Understanding and Responding to Self-Harm: The One-Stop Guide

Allan House is Professor of Liaison Psychiatry at Leeds Institute of Health Sciences in the School of Medicine. He first came to Leeds to work in clinical practice as a consultant in the NHS and now spends most of his time researching and teaching in the University of Leeds. He has co-authored many academic papers on self-harm and is currently researching new approaches to helping people who repeatedly self-harm.

Other titles in the 'One-Stop Guide' series

Understanding and Responding to Self-Harm: The One-Stop Guide

Practical advice for anybody affected by self-harm

Allan House

PROFILE BOOKS

First published in Great Britain in 2019 by
PROFILE BOOKS LTD
3 Holford Yard
Bevin Way
London
WC1X 9HD

www.profilebooks.com

The advice and recommendations given in this book are provided
in good faith, but no responsibility for any consequences, however
caused, of acting on them will be accepted by the author or the
publisher. If in doubt, seek suitable advice from a healthcare
professional.

A CIP catalogue record for this book is available from the
British Library.

ISBN 978 1 78816 027 8
eISBN: 978 1 78283 435 9

Designed by *sue@lambledesign.demon.co.uk*
Typeset in Dante by MacGuru Ltd
Printed and bound by CPI Group (UK) Ltd, Croydon CR0 4YY

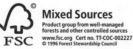

Contents

Introduction

It's not difficult to find things to read about self-harm in magazines, books or on social media – it's a topic that seems to attract attention from all sections of society. That's no surprise really. With more than one in five young people reporting that they have self-harmed at some time, it is something that will have touched the lives of most of us – whether we've done it ourselves or are the friends or families of those who have.

The trouble is that what you can read about self-harm is not always helpful. Film stars who talk about it can make it sound like a lifestyle choice. Melodramatic accounts of self-harm in the lives of mass murderers make it sound like a symptom of deep disturbance. Gloom-laden stories about suicide in young people touch on an important topic, but sometimes they seem designed to cause shock and dismay rather than to help our understanding of the problem and what we can do about it.

What is harder to find is a simple account of what self-harm is, what we know about its causes, and what you can do to seek or offer help. It is this gap that this book aims to fill, by offering clear and sound advice.

The book covers some important topics – including what self-harm is and the reasons for it. It seeks to explain the apparent contradiction that self-harm isn't the same as attempted suicide and yet the person doing it may be suicidal. Self-harm isn't something that only young people do, or only women, and it certainly isn't something that people just do for attention. I will look at the role of social media and whether it's true that it makes self-harm in young people more likely. You may have read about self-harm and people with so-called personality disorder – an idea that has broken through into popular journalism – 'What to do if your partner has borderline personality disorder' and so on. I'll explain what this term means, and discuss what psychiatry has to offer in more useful ways than attaching labels to people. And most importantly this book will challenge the idea that you can't do anything about self-harm – it is possible to help.

In writing this book I have drawn heavily on my own experience over many years of talking to people who have self-harmed and to others who have approached me for advice about somebody they are concerned about. For fifteen years, I worked as a consultant in a busy hospital-based self-harm service in which we saw many hundreds of people each year, and both the users of our service and the staff I worked with taught me much.

Throughout this book you will find quotes from people who have self-harmed, descriptions of people and their problems, and brief boxed 'case studies'. All these accounts are based upon real people, but I have made sure of confidentiality by changing names and some of the personal details so that nobody can be identified.

As well as being a psychiatrist, I am also an academic and researcher, and so what I have to say in this book is based not just on my personal and professional experience but also upon research, some of it mine, much of it by others.

I wrote this book with a wide audience in mind – people who have harmed themselves and those who live with them, care about them or support them, and people who work in roles that bring them into contact with self-harm: in fact, anybody with a genuine interest, perhaps a little knowledge, and a desire to understand the topic more deeply. It saddens me to hear how often someone who self-harms has sought help and yet not found it easy to get. Those close to them have responded with shock, dismay, anger or panic and haven't known what to do. Professionals have been apparently uninterested or unable to offer anything. And yet my experience is that many people do want to help – they just don't understand the problem and don't know what to do about it. This book is also for them.

This book can be read cover to cover, but I know that many people don't read like that, so each chapter can be read on its own. That occasionally requires a little repetition, which I have tried to keep to the minimum required to make each chapter stand alone.

You may find some of what I have to say about what people do and why they do it quite direct – I think it is important to be clear in describing and discussing the issues. I hope you do not find any of the detail too upsetting, and above all I hope you find what I have to say informative and, more importantly, helpful.

part one

What is self-harm?

chapter 1

What do we mean by 'self-harm'?

If you are trying to find out about self-harm (especially by looking online) you can end up muddled by what seem to be contradictory statements. Or you may read something about self-harm and think 'that's all very well but it doesn't apply to me' even though you yourself self-harm or know somebody who does. Of course, self-harm is an emotive topic and that is partly why the way in which people talk about it gets muddled. Another reason is that the expression 'self-harm' isn't used at all consistently. So, to avoid confusion, let's start by examining what self-harm is, and exploring how different terms are used by different people. On the way, we will also debunk some of the myths that surround the topic.

Defining 'self-harm': keep it broad and keep it simple

WHO, the World Health Organization, issues definitions of illnesses and conditions. The WHO defines self-harm as

an act with non-fatal outcome, in which an

individual deliberately initiates a non-habitual behaviour that, without intervention from others, will cause self-harm, or deliberately ingests a substance in excess of the prescribed or generally recognised therapeutic dosage, and which is aimed at realising changes which the subject desired via the actual or expected physical consequences.

That definition means that self-harm is intentional, is done by somebody to themselves, and is done by someone who wants to make something change. By saying it is 'non-habitual' it means that it is done as a conscious act, separate from normal day-to-day life.

The WHO definition might seem a bit mind-boggling and rather legalistic-sounding, so here's a simpler one, adopted by the UK's National Institute for Health and Clinical Excellence (usually called NICE): 'self-poisoning or self-injury, irrespective of the apparent purpose of the act'.

That is the definition of self-harm used in this book. Let's look in a bit of detail about what it means in practice.

First and foremost, self-harm is an action by a person. It's something that somebody does to themselves. It is not a description of who somebody is and not a name for a mental disorder. You sometimes hear people described as 'cutters' or 'self-harmers'. That's undesirable language and it's offensive. It is dismissive to label someone because of something they do. Even if they do it quite often it doesn't define them as a person. And as a description of their actions it's misleading because it is oversimplified. Even if we do something over and over, it does not mean that our actions are unchanging and fixed.

You will notice that neither of these definitions says anything about the reasons that the person has for their act of self-harm. You have to remember that the definitions include acts of attempted suicide but also acts where there is no apparent desire to die. The definitions also include those times when the person actively rejects any notion that they wanted or intended to die. This is an important point. Ever since the 1950s, when self-harm started to be seen as a common problem in developed countries, it has been clear that every act of self-harm is not a failed attempt at suicide.

As will be discussed later when I review explanations for self-harm, some people are quite clear that they don't want to die at the time they harm themselves. They may in fact be using non-fatal self-harm as a way of defending themselves against more threatening thoughts about suicide. On the other hand, self-harm is definitely not the opposite of attempted suicide. Some non-fatal acts are indeed failed suicide attempts. And research studies that have followed large groups of people who had already harmed themselves find that they have a suicide rate many times higher than the rest of the population.

To summarise, whatever definition is used, the reasons for self-harm are complicated and in truth many people find it difficult to put into words exactly why they have harmed themselves. They may or may not intend to die. Some may eventually die through self-harm. Nevertheless, the person you know who has self-harmed may actually have reduced the likelihood of their suicide by resorting to a harmful but not fatal act. The most important point to make is this: when someone has self-harmed, you can't make any assumption about whether or not they intended to kill themselves. It isn't wise to make blanket assumptions.

Before we move on, here are a few other terms that you may come across. *Self-harm* and *deliberate self-harm* are used to mean the same thing. They can be regarded as identical, although *self-harm* is now more commonly used. *Parasuicide* is an expression that isn't used so much now, but you might find it in older writings. It's a word that was made up in the 1960s to mean 'behaviour that's like suicidal behaviour'. It has (not surprisingly) fallen out of fashion. *Attempted suicide* sounds as if it refers only to acts where death was desired, but in fact it was quite widely used from the 1970s onwards to refer to all acts of self-harm. *Self-mutilation* is really the same as self-injury, and has been dropped as a term in most settings. This is because 'mutilation' means disfigurement or maiming, and a lot of self-injury isn't deliberately intended to cause that sort of injury, or permanent scars. Sometimes, even if there is such an intention, there is in fact no permanent effect.

When self-damaging actions aren't called self-harm

There are lots of harmful things people do to their

bodies that don't usually get counted as 'self-harm' in the sense I am talking about. Here are some of the common ones:

- Piercing the body for fashionable (cosmetic) reasons
- Cutting patterns on the body for social or symbolic reasons (scarification)
- Taking dietary modification to extremes – undertaking prolonged fasts or excluding all but an extremely limited number of foods from the diet
- Using recreational drugs or alcohol in a wild or reckless manner.

Why aren't these activities usually included in the category of self-harm? One reason is that their primary purpose isn't to damage the body. For example, several of the actions in this list are designed to change the body's physical appearance for social or cultural reasons that are seen as desirable rather than damaging – even when taken to extremes as in prolonged starvation such as anorexia nervosa. Bodily damage, including serious illness, can arise from drinking too much or taking recreational drugs, but the primary purpose of using these substances is to experience their psychological effects rather than to cause damage. So, these are sometimes called *indirectly harmful behaviours* to distinguish them from the intentionally harmful actions that are labelled as self-harm.

The other reason that these activities are talked about differently is that they are thought of as being socially approved – that is, shared and supported within a social group – whereas self-harm is thought of as having individual and abnormal psychological causes.

As with all simple distinctions, it isn't that straightforward. There is in reality a rather unclear boundary between actions where damage to yourself is an unintended consequence and acts of self-harm where damage is intended. For example, studies into how young people respond to stress have shown that self-harm, drinking too much and eating disorders may often go together. It is also possible that someone who regularly uses substances in a way that their social group tolerates may push themselves beyond the 'normal' range for that group.

Acts that are definitely in the category of self-harm – cutting your arms to produce scars – can sometimes be so common as to seem normal in certain social groups that aim for a rebellious image. This particular example shows that apparently simple distinctions can be less clear than they seem initially.

Do people who engage in indirectly harmful behaviours for unhealthy reasons, or who self-harm for reasons accepted by a group to which they belong, need protection against doing harm to themselves? There is no simple answer to these questions, especially when talking about young people. It is an active debate in public health. For now, these issues have been raised in order to clarify that in this book self-harm is referring only to intentionally harmful actions.

So far this chapter has outlined what professionals mean when they use the expression 'self-harm'. It isn't how everybody uses the expression, but it is a helpful and simple way – it doesn't make the idea too broad by including too many different behaviours, and yet it doesn't narrow it down too much by (for example) limiting it to only one method of self-harm or one presumed motive.

It can be difficult to know what definitions mean without clear examples, so the next section will look at what self-harm is by going into more detail about what people actually do. Not every possibility is described, but it will cover all the common methods of self-harm.

Describing self-harm – what people do

The definition of self-harm by the World Health Organization refers to 'a non-habitual behaviour' or acts in which somebody 'deliberately ingests a substance in excess of the prescribed or generally recognised therapeutic dosage'. The NICE definition more concisely describes the two main types of self-harm as 'self-poisoning or self-injury'.

One of the confusions you come across in the use of language is that some people use the term self-harm to refer only to self-injury. For example if you put 'self-harm' into an internet search engine you get lots of material (especially if you search for images) about people who cut themselves. It is almost as if people who poison themselves aren't thought of as self-harming, or as if they are completely different from people who self-injure. Commonly, an act of self-poisoning is likely to be seen as attempted suicide while self-cutting is seen as non-suicidal. Indeed the label 'non-suicidal self-injury', which is widely used especially in the US, suggests exactly this distinction. It's true that people who self-harm a lot, perhaps dozens of times a year, are likely to use self-cutting most of the time but we shouldn't think of these two acts (cutting and poisoning) as being completely different. There is plenty of evidence that this way of thinking – about self-harm being exclusively the same as self-injury while self-poisoning is something different – is wrong. Self-poisoning and self-injury have pretty much the same causes, both can be associated with thoughts of wanting to die or can take place with no wish to die at the time, and people who repeatedly self-harm will often switch between self-injury and self-poisoning as their chosen method.

There are a couple of reasons why self-injury attracts so much attention. First, we live in a very 'visual' world and it's easier to show pictures of somebody with scars or holding a razor blade than it is of somebody taking an overdose of tablets. Second, some of the interest in self-injury comes from a sort of horrified fascination with it – 'How could anybody do that to themselves?'

A balanced view of self-harm requires us to consider *all* its aspects. So, let's start by reviewing both self-poisoning *and* self-injury.

Self-poisoning

If you work in a hospital, the commonest type of self-harm you see is self-poisoning – often called an overdose because what people typically do is to swallow too much of readily available prescribed or over-the-counter medications. The common ones that people take are physical painkillers (paracetamol, aspirin, ibuprofen) or medications for emotional pain, such as tranquillisers or antidepressants.

I felt so awful, I just wanted it to stop, to switch off for a while. I went into the bathroom cupboard and found some tablets of my mum's – painkillers her doctor gave her when she injured her back. There was 10 left in the pack, it said the adult dose was two so I took them all and lay down in my bedroom.

Laura, 19

Less commonly, poisoning can be with substances that have no value as medication – for example bleach or household products that are poisonous. The choice of poison may depend upon its availability. In agricultural communities weed killer is more widely used. Powerful painkillers that are like morphine (called opioids) are usually only available on prescription and are more often used in urban areas. You may have read that this problem of opioid prescribing and the risk in overdose is a public health concern now in the US, where they are facing a sharp rise in both non-fatal overdose and of suicides with these drugs. It is less of a problem in the UK, where doctors are increasingly discouraged from prescribing strong painkillers for people unless they have a life-limiting physical illness like cancer.

Self-injury

Most acts of self-harm do not lead to hospital

attendance, and in these cases it is self-injury that is the more frequent method used. Here are some of the ways in which people injure themselves:

Cutting with razors, broken glass, knives – anything sharp enough

Self-cutting is such a pervasive act now that nearly everybody will have heard of it or will know somebody who has done it. Most commonly, it is obviously accessible parts of the body that people cut – the forearms and thighs – but other body parts are also targets, such as the abdomen, upper arms and (for women) on or under the breasts.

What do people actually do when they cut themselves? For some it is an impulsive act, carried out without much planning or forethought:

Mike told me about the last time he cut himself: 'I went out to the pub with a couple of mates from work. We had a few drinks and chatted about the usual things – football, what we planned for the weekend. We didn't leave that late and separated to go our own ways home. Walking along the street it suddenly came to me how alone I was and how bad I felt about myself. Just at that moment I saw a bottle standing in a doorway; I smashed it and cut into my arm while I was standing there.'

Melanie, community psychiatric nurse

On the other hand, some cutting is planned and thought about for a while beforehand:

I always know when I am going to cut myself. I think about it during the day and anticipate being on my own in my room in the evening, when I'll be able to do it without being disturbed. I keep a blade in my room and a bandage in case I need to do something to stop bleeding.

Anna, 26

How people cut themselves varies hugely. Cuts can be single or multiple; they may always be made in the same part of the body or made in different places all over the body. Multiple acts can look as if they are made at random or they can form obvious patterns in rows or grids. This patterned cutting can look so organised and carefully planned that you might wonder if the person was really that upset when they did it. The answer is that all self-harm is a sign of distress, even when it isn't physically damaging – you should never be dismissive about it and even when you don't understand it you should take it seriously. I'll say more about this later. Sometimes people write words on their skin – usually self-critical words.

Sarah was alone in her bedroom brooding about her life and especially about an argument at school that confirmed in her view that she was unpopular and that the teachers thought she was a second-rater who would never do much with her life. She fiddled with a razor blade for five minutes and then scratched 'loser' in the skin on her forearm. She felt she deserved the pain it caused and that other people would think so too.

Child psychiatrist

Burning, with cigarettes, matches, candles

Here I am not thinking necessarily about people who set themselves on fire. That is a very rare event. Much more frequently, when used as a form of self-harm, burning seems very like cutting in that it produces an instantaneous quite localised injury that is painful. Examples include stubbing out cigarettes on the body, or holding a match or candle to the skin.

Sticking pins or needles into the body

Unlike the methods of self-injury noted above, sticking pins or needles into the body may leave no external mark. Medical problems arise if the needle slips in too far so that it can't be removed without surgical intervention. Most commonly this injury is inflicted by sticking needles into the abdomen or breasts.

Punching walls, head banging

Although these are sometimes things that people do when they are angry or frustrated – to get it out of their system rather than to cause injury – hitting yourself against a hard object can be a way of causing self-injury that looks accidental.

Jane was at home when she pulled a door hard towards herself so that it hit her in the face. When her parents came home they noticed the bruising and she told them she had fallen in the street and hadn't been able to put a hand out to break her fall.

Helen, high school counsellor

Other distressed behaviours

There are some acts that can be quite difficult to judge. Are they forms of self-harm or are they ways of communicating distress? For example, wading into or jumping into water, or tying ligatures round the neck. They may not lead to an injury and if other people are around they may not be very risky. On the other hand drowning and hanging are both well-known methods of suicide. Another example is walking into busy traffic.

Maria was picked up by the police following a call from a worried motorist who had swerved to avoid her moments earlier, as she walked in the middle of a busy two-lane city road. She was taken to a place of safety by the police and interviewed there by a member of the duty mental health team. She said she didn't care if she lived or died, although it was reported that she hadn't actively tried to throw herself in front of a moving vehicle.

Actually, this example shows the limitations of definitions. Maria was doing something that signals a need for careful assessment and help, and her actions could easily have led to serious injury. You will remember that the World Health Organization definition included acts that ' … without intervention from others, will cause self-harm … '. So, our definition of self-harm includes all acts regardless of intention. It does not limit the use of the term to describe particular methods of self-harm or even to acts that have definitely led to self-harm, only to ones that could have done without intervention.

Mixing methods of self-harm

Although most acts of self-harm involve *either* poisoning *or* self-injury, sometimes people do both at the same time. This is a common finding in studies of attendances in hospital emergency departments. In about 5 per cent (one in twenty) of attendances, the person who has self-harmed has self-poisoned and self-injured at the same time. For example, it isn't at all rare for healthcare staff to meet people who have taken an overdose and cut themselves as part of the same episode.

Furthermore, in research, if we follow up a group of people who have contacted hospital services after an episode of self-harm, what we find is that quite a lot of them (about a quarter, in fact) will harm themselves again within a year. What is less well known is that many of these repeat acts use a different method; that is, somebody seen after an episode of self-cutting is quite likely, the next time they present to hospital, to have taken an overdose.

It is for these reasons – because some people use both methods of self-harm at the same time, and because people who repeat self-harm quite often switch method – that it's important to keep an open mind about what defines self-harm.

It's for the same reason that you shouldn't confuse individuals with methods. Talking about 'cutters', for example, would make you focus on *what* a person did on the occasion that they harmed themselves rather than asking *why*. It is more important to see past the method, to the person with a particular problem. They might turn up on another occasion having hurt themselves in a different way, or they may have done something different before. Labels are not helpful, especially when you remember that people who self-harm are more likely than others to die from suicide. They stigmatise the person rather than offering understanding of how to help them.

And here is one more observation about how using so many terms to describe self-harm can lead to muddle. In 2018, many newspapers reported that one in four teenage girls said that they had self-harmed. One article was accompanied by a story about a young woman who had been cutting herself since she was 13 years old. The implication was that this was the sort of thing that all these girls were doing. However, the reports did not say what question had been asked, or how the answers had been judged. Suppose the question was 'Have you ever done anything to harm yourself?' and the girls had answered 'Yes' if they had ever fallen over when drunk, or had deliberately made themselves sick, or had taken a drug in a club that made them ill. In that case it would be misleading to link the figure of one in four to the story about repeated self-cutting. This is just one example of the ways in which reporting can obscure the nature of self-harm.

Is self-harm always serious?

It doesn't seem right to suggest that *any* act of self-harm is trivial. Surely anybody who is moved to try to do harm to themselves has a serious problem in some sense? On the other hand, some acts are particularly worrying. They seem to need a more urgent response, and may be a sign of additional major problems for the person involved. So by understanding the seriousness of the action we can come to a better understanding of the person we are thinking about, and also make decisions about what we should do to help.

In determining whether or not an act of self-harm is serious, we can begin by saying that 'seriousness' might be defined in different ways. That is, the act may be serious in any of three ways – physically, socially or psychologically. So if we are trying to make sense of a particular act of self-harm – whether as a friend or family member or as a professional, we might ask three questions, as follows.

Question 1: Is the act of self-harm physically serious?

One way to judge the seriousness of self-harm is to look at the physical severity of the damage done. In self-poisoning that may not be obvious from the outside, and so the best course of action is always to take someone to hospital for assessment.

In self-poisoning the damage caused can be immediate – for example, swallowing strong chemicals can cause instant damage to the throat or stomach. The

warning labels and special containers for these substances advertise what effects they can have. Taking
drugs like heroin or barbiturates in overdose is
extremely dangerous because they suppress breathing.
Here it is worth noting that alcohol is involved with
many acts of self-poisoning. Lots of people have been
drinking either just beforehand or as part of swallowing
other substances. Since alcohol itself can also suppress
breathing, it is especially dangerous when taken in
combination with an overdose of a sedating drug.

Self-poisoning can also lead to delayed damage to
the organs of your body. Probably the best-known
example is the liver damage caused by paracetamol,
which typically starts early but builds up over days
after the tablets have been taken. The person, having
taken the drugs, may present themselves at a hospital
for treatment when they aren't too ill, only to become
increasingly sick, deteriorating over several days.

The physical seriousness of self-poisoning is influenced not just by the type of poison swallowed but
by the amount taken – for example by the number of
tablets of a prescribed medication taken.

Realisation that some medications are dangerous
in even small doses has led doctors to work to elimi-
nate certain drugs altogether from their prescribing:
two examples are barbiturates and the sedating drug
chlormethiazole (Heminevrin). These were widely
used until recently but have largely disappeared since
doctors reduced prescribing in response to increased
awareness of the risks of misuse. A painkiller like
paracetamol isn't quite so dangerous in small doses,

and recent legislation has mandated that packs contain only a few tablets and that only a limited number of tablets can be bought in a single purchase. The result is that the number of serious overdoses of the drug now being seen in hospitals has been reduced.

The same question can be asked of self-injury, that is: how physically injurious is it? The severity of most injuries can be judged visually, just as you would if you cut yourself accidentally. More severe-looking injuries merit careful examination by a professional, to check on possible damage to sensitive parts of the body like nerves and blood vessels. The injuries people inflict can vary greatly. At one end of the spectrum, self-injury can involve light scratches that don't bleed and heal quickly without scarring. Sometimes people make multiple light scratches like this. There has formerly been a tendency to be dismissive about this scratching. However, it's worth bearing in mind the common observation that superficial cuts can be considerably more painful than sharp deep cuts, and that the person who self-injures in this way may be putting themselves through much greater pain over a long period of time, suffering for longer, and feeling even more stressed and constrained to keep their psychological and physical pain secret.

Not all cuts are slight. Injuries that require bandaging or suturing are common, and at other times cuts can be so deep that surgery is needed to repair tendons or blood vessels in order to avoid damage from loss of blood supply to a limb, permanent paralysis from nerve damage, loss of sensation, or further complications such as scarring that limits movements. Many people who cut themselves do not go to hospital afterwards, usually because they are worried about the reaction of staff. However, if a wound is deep it really is a good idea to have it checked out to make sure that it is safe or to prevent infection, for example. And early careful management can reduce later scarring.

Question 2: Is the act of self-harm socially serious?

This may seem like an odd question but it makes the point that part of the seriousness of self-harm lies in its intrusiveness or impact on day-to-day life. That is, even if self-harm isn't very severe in the physical injury it causes it can be serious in terms of the effect it has on somebody's ability to live a full life.

One clue to the likely impact of self-harm is the frequency with which acts are occurring. If self-harm suggests (as it does) that the person doing it is troubled, then repeated self-harm suggests a person in deep trouble who is unable to see a way of using their personal and social resources to get out of that trouble. Repeated self-harm can be an isolating and preoccupying experience that makes it difficult to live a full life with other people. It is therefore ironic that repeated self-harm can lead to people being taken *less* seriously, as if something you keep doing can't be that important.

Many people who harm themselves will only do so once or perhaps twice in their lives. Typically, the self-harm occurs in the middle of an emotional crisis that temporarily overwhelms someone's ability to cope. With time and help, an individual can get back on top of their problems and the distress they cause, and self-harm becomes a thing of the past.

However, that isn't always the case. Nobody knows the figures for sure, but a small proportion of those who harm themselves will do it several times, and an even smaller proportion will do it many, many times – in extreme cases nearly every day. I'll come to why that might be later on but for now, note that frequency by itself is a serious sign. This is irrespective of the physical severity of the act of self-harm. The person who does it is likely to be struggling to lead a satisfying life, and struggling to hold on to satisfactory relationships with others. Even people who self-harm repeatedly can and do stop in time, so one shouldn't assume that repeated episodes are a sign that things will never change.

Question 3: Is the act of self-harm psychologically (personally) serious?

No doubt, self-harm is a personal act and driven by personal motives. If we accept that doing harm to yourself is a bad idea, a sign that the person who does it is troubled, then the seriousness of the self-harm may be judged by how serious are the psychological or emotional issues lying behind it. We will cover much of this ground in later parts of the book about reasons for self-harm.

Research shows that knowing how serious an act is in physical or social terms does not tell you much about how serious it is psychologically. You can't judge it by the size of the injury, or how life-threatening it is or how much it interferes with somebody's relationships. One reason for this is that people don't always realise how much harm they might do in an episode because they don't understand their body or how it works, or the effects of medications. Imagine these two scenarios:

◆ First think of a man who feels hopeless about life and wants to die; he takes all of his wife's sleeping tablets (there are fifteen in the bottle) expecting not to wake up. But in fact the tablets are extremely safe in overdose (many sleeping tablets are) and he wakes up in hospital the next day having been discovered by his family. The act was not physically serious but it is a marker of something very serious in his mental state.

◆ In a different scenario, imagine a young teenager who takes an angry overdose of her mother's tablets after a row with her mother about the friends she is keeping. Unfortunately, the tablets are for a heart problem and the girl develops life-threatening complications. The act is extremely serious physically but reflects a passing emotional state and may not therefore be very psychologically significant. How serious it is socially depends on the background relationship with her parents and the reason she felt the desire to express anger at her mother's attitude to her friends.

The point is that it isn't possible to judge the nature of what is going on simply by looking at the act itself.

Self-harm, as defined in this chapter, is really common. More than one in five young people say that they have done it at some time in their lives. In the

NHS, at least 120,000 people each year go to hospital for treatment after an act of self-harm. For every 1,000 adults living in the UK, something like 40 to 50 will harm themselves each year.

Although a great deal of attention in the media is given to self-harm caused by repeated cutting, that isn't the only type of self-harm seen in practice. In hospital practice about three quarters of those who come for treatment have poisoned themselves. And although repeated self-harm is common, over half those who go to hospital after self-harm won't do it again. Only about one in ten will keep repeating the act.

A family member or friend needs to encourage the person who has self-harmed to get a proper assessment. You can ask for this for yourself, through your GP or by contacting other helping groups (for examples, see the list of resources at the end of this book). It is important to know that other people do this, and that they have had help and have found other ways of dealing with what is troubling them. You may feel hopeless or afraid, but the first step is a proper assessment. Later in this book there is a list of organisations that can help.

A proper assessment requires asking questions about all three of these areas: the physical seriousness of the act (actual and intended); the social consequences of self-harm and the context in which it occurs (how disrupted and poorly functioning relationships are); and what emotional and psychological problems lie behind the act and motivate it.

In the next chapter I'll talk a bit more about why people self-harm by considering who it affects.

part two

Why do people self-harm?

chapter 2

What we know about who self-harms

At times, self-harm seems to be everywhere. It's portrayed in TV soap operas and in popular films and drama series, written about in magazines and talked about by celebrities. It's not difficult to find personal accounts posted on blogs and other social media outlets and news items appear regularly in all outlets.

This high-profile portrayal isn't much help if we don't understand why self-harm happens. So, what do we really know about why people self-harm? If we can answer that question – and that's what we'll try to do in the next three chapters – then we'll be a long way towards being able to find ways to help.

This chapter considers who self-harms, how common it is and whether it's really getting more common in certain groups. The study of these general patterns in society is called epidemiology when it relates to health-related problems, and can tell us something important about reasons for all sorts of conditions.

In the UK, there are three main sources of information that help us answer this question about population patterns of self-harm.

First, and longest established, there are reports from

NHS services that give information about people who go for treatment after self-harm – not their identities or personal information, but their general characteristics. Most of these studies have been based upon hospital attendances, especially in the emergency department, although recent studies have also reported on contacts made in general practice. Recently in the UK headlines have been made by such reports, which showed that self-harm rates had increased dramatically among teenage girls. The statistics behind these reports came from an official body, now called NHS Digital, which collects statistics about hospital attendance. The figures also come from GP computerised records. These figures are interesting and usually quite accurate, but they are limited because they only tell us about people who have gone to a doctor for help – either with their mental health problems or for the physical effects of what they have done. So we need other sources of information.

A second source of information comes from the results of large-scale surveys like the National Psychiatric Morbidity Survey and the National Household Survey, which are funded by government and cover many topics of which one is self-harm. These surveys have the advantage that they allow us to estimate how common self-harm is in the general population, counting even those of us who don't consult a doctor at all about what we have done. Their main disadvantage is that they rely on self-reporting from the people surveyed so they may not be very accurate – not surprisingly some people will not want to tell an official survey about an episode of self-harm that they have previously kept to themselves. Also, memory – even for something as important as self-harm – may be unreliable, and we can all forget events, especially, perhaps, those that we'd rather not remember.

Our third source of information about self-harm is academic research studies, and especially those aimed at identifying people who self-harm but don't present to health services for help. This has been an important source of information about, for example, self-harm in young people of school age. Some studies have surveyed classes in school, hoping to get a complete 'catch' of children of a certain age. Others have been based on what are called birth cohorts – following everybody born at a certain time and place as they grow up. These studies have the same advantage as national government surveys and the same disadvantage – the replies don't depend on somebody having sought help but they may be influenced by reluctance to confide in the person asking the questions. And cohort studies have the additional disadvantage of losing contact with individuals as the years go by.

So, all our sources of information have some disadvantages but they still provide a reasonable picture of what is happening.

The first thing we can say with some confidence is that a lot of people who harm themselves don't go and see either their GP or a hospital doctor about it. I spoke to a colleague, who is a consultant in one of the two acute hospitals in Leeds, about the picture locally (Leeds has a population of about three quarters of a million). She told me:

About ten people come each day to one of the two Leeds hospitals after an episode of self-harm, and over the twelve months after a hospital visit we know that about a quarter of those individuals will come back again after another episode. But we also know that there are as many people again who are harming themselves at home and not coming for help – managing the consequences of what they have done on their own.

With any other health problem people don't always seek professional help, and it's the same with self-harm. And we can be reluctant to answer questions about sensitive topics – how much we drink, for example, or our sexual behaviour – even when asked by somebody who promises confidentiality: and this is also the case for self-harm. As a result, what we know from all this research is that the picture we have of self-harm is incomplete and, perhaps, not very accurate.

All the same, the information that we have is better than nothing and that's why it is worth discussing. But remember that it's incomplete, and that's one reason that you may not recognise your own problems in what you read about self-harm. Let's look at what we do know.

Age and gender

Self-harm is very rare before puberty. It's more and more common after that, peaking in frequency in the early twenties and then getting less and less common. However, it is important not to think of it solely as a problem of young people: a quarter of those who come to hospital after an episode of self-harm are aged over 40.

No one knows exactly why self-harm gets less common in later life. Maybe it's because life settles down and offers fewer challenges as we get older. It's probably also something to do with people finding different ways to respond to stressful circumstances as age brings experience. For example, you may have seen in the news that there is a worry about mental health problems and self-harm among young people who are studying at university. Although university life is privileged in some ways it is stressful in others – finding somewhere to live isn't always that easy, money can be tight, making new relationships may be fun, but also daunting. Suddenly in a different world from the one you grew up in, you may have to ask yourself where you sit in the social pecking order, if you are cool or not, how many friends you have. And at the same time you are away from home, perhaps for the first time, and you may be reluctant to share problems with old friends or family who have expectations of you making a success of your studies. These are problems that, by middle life, most people will have met and dealt with before so they have a fund of experience – their own and that of those close to them – that they can bring to bear on finding solutions.

A striking feature of self-harm is its relationship with gender. When self-harm first becomes common after puberty it is much more common among girls and young women; at the ages of 12 to 14 or so, girls outnumber boys by two or three to one. Over the next few years the genders balance out a bit so that by the late twenties and onwards there really isn't much difference between men and women in how often they self-harm. Of course some of this might initially be because girls reach puberty earlier than boys but the differences are too large and too persistent for that to be the only explanation.

Why are girls and young women more prone to self-harm than boys and young men? The explanations are more likely to be linked to life problems rather than to the different physical make-up of boys and girls. Girls may have more stresses in their early teens than boys do, and they certainly tend to have different types of stress. Even if the amount of stress is similar for both boys and girls, gender is often associated with different ways of responding to it. Young men are more likely to get into trouble with alcohol misuse, drug abuse or difficulties with the law. Young women, perhaps because they are bombarded with messages about appearance throughout their lives, are more likely to express distress in a bodily way – developing eating disorders or harming themselves. These different ways of responding to stress aren't hard-wired as part of the biological difference between the sexes. They are picked up throughout life, as more or less accepted ways of 'being' male or female – in our families, among our friends and in our wider social world. Of course young men do also self-harm, often for the same reasons, but sometimes for different reasons too (see Chapter 10 for more about self-harm and gender).

There's another aspect of gender that is important in relation to self-harm, and that is what our sense is of our own gender identity: that is, what we think ourselves about whether we are truly male, female or something less specifically or traditionally defined. This sense of gender identity can be a real cause of distress for a couple of reasons. First, if you aren't clear about, or are unhappy with, your gender, it can make your whole life feel unsettled and uncertain. Second, even if you are certain about your gender it can be a real worry if your own sense of gender doesn't match your bodily characteristics – not least a worry because of fears about what others may think of you. We know that self-harm is common among people with these dilemmas, and also that it is hard to seek help when you feel like this. If worries about gender or sexuality affect you, it really is important that you try to find somebody you can trust to confide in – it's not something you should have to struggle with on your own.

In the last three or four decades, rates of self-harm among young people have increased to be three to four times what they were. Life may be more stressful, but not that much more stressful. What has happened is that for young men and young women, self-harm has become a socially understood way of responding to stress in a way that it wasn't a couple of generations ago.

Personal circumstances and self-harm

Rather obviously, you can't understand self-harm just by knowing a few facts about somebody, such as how old they are, their gender, and so on; you need to know something about the life they are living. Indeed, if you ask someone who has self-harmed about it, they will almost certainly tell you a story about their personal circumstances. Here are some of the common features of those stories.

◆ *Difficulty in relationships* – either in the family or in friendship or romantic relationships. Tension and arguments are a common part of the problem, perhaps associated with violence and sometimes made worse by the unhealthy use of alcohol. Such difficulty may be long-standing and amount at times to abuse, or it may be more recent and represent a change.

◆ *Loss in relationships* – romantic relationships, partnerships and marriages can break up. Even when a relationship was going badly a sense of loss can follow a break-up, along with anxieties about the future. Bereavement can carry with it the additional burden of losing a trusted source of emotional and practical support – if a close friend dies, for example, or a parent.

◆ *Practical problems* – Self-harm is so often seen as a response to emotional and psychological troubles that it is easy to forget how frequently practical problems are a part of what weighs people down. Financial difficulties and debt, housing problems, unemployment and so on are real and are associated with genuine distress. They often feature in stories about self-harm, particularly in the current period that has seen cuts in the welfare state, something that has affected many people. The stress of all this is of course practical but it is also emotional – because of the double message that you aren't going to get the support you need and that society doesn't much care about the consequences.

◆ *Physical illness and disability* – one of the greatest threats we face is that of physical illness and, in cases of chronic illness, of disability. Physical illness is particularly difficult to live with when it is associated with symptoms such as chronic pain. It may also bring with it some of the practical problems noted above but it also threatens our status, in both our personal lives and in society.

I suppose I just thought it would never happen to me. When you're young, you know you don't think about it – as if you're immortal. Not being able to see properly is the worst and [starts crying] not being able to pick up my baby granddaughter and play with her …

Alice, 74

◆ *Sex and sexuality* – it may be true that sex isn't everything in life, but it is still an important part of life for many people. We have generally become more tolerant of the diversity of human interests in this area and that is to be welcomed, but it is still true that living a happy sex life can be a real challenge for some people. This is perhaps especially true for those who are struggling with uncertainty about their sexual orientation, or those who are happy with their sexuality but are unsure about how to confide in those close to them. Bullying or abuse is still, unfortunately, part of the experience of many whose sexual orientation is not exclusively heterosexual, and under those circumstances it is easy to feel excluded or threatened and isolated.

John told me that he knew he'd been gay since he was 13 but hadn't been able to come out. He'd tried going out with girls but had avoided relationships that might become physical. He was athletic in build and played in a local football team where he enjoyed the sport but was uncomfortable with the laddish social atmosphere and tolerance of homophobic banter. At the same time, he didn't like what he described to me as the 'camp silliness' of a gay bar he went to once (in another town to avoid being recognised). He didn't feel he belonged anywhere.

There are as many ways of describing personal circumstances as there are people, and if what troubles you hasn't been mentioned in this list it is not because it's unimportant. The list is intended to point to some common aspects of the stories people tell to explain their self-harm and to emphasise just how varied those stories are.

This isn't to say that personal circumstances are enough to explain self-harm. Many people who live with these problems don't self-harm so there must be more to the explanation.

Individual characteristics and self-harm

In this chapter, we are looking at the personal side of self-harm: the *who* rather than the *what*. Let's turn now to the idea that people who have certain individual or psychological characteristics are more likely to harm themselves.

If you ask somebody who has harmed themselves recently why they did it, they very commonly describe a stressful occurrence or experience. Someone has treated them badly, either recently or in the past; a relationship has broken down; or there are pressing practical or financial worries. These sound like good reasons to be distressed: are some people more likely than others to express that distress by self-harm?

One answer might be: 'No, it's not so much about the individual as it is about their circumstances.' For example, self-harm is more common in certain environments such as prisons, and particularly in women's prisons. It's not difficult to understand the reasons for this – prisoners have more than the average amount of personal and social difficulty, and being locked up reduces their ability to cope in ways that they might do outside. Drug misuse is extremely common in prisons: it's tempting because of easy access to illicit drugs and there are few other ways to deal with distress. So we can understand a lot about high rates of self-harm in some settings simply by knowing about the stresses that those settings cause, without needing to say that there's something different about the people who do it.

Even so, we know that not everybody responds to

the same set of circumstances in the same way, so it seems likely that there are individual explanations for why some people self-harm when stressed while others don't. What might those individual differences be? Below, we'll look at four possible answers to this question: first, whether people who self-harm have certain ways of thinking about themselves or their problems; second, whether they are more prone to other types of destructive actions as well as self-harm; third, whether people who self-harm are more likely to have a psychiatric disorder; and finally, whether people with one type of personality are more likely to self-harm.

Ways of thinking and self-harm

What about the idea that self-harm is more common among people who have certain styles of thinking? We all have particular ways of thinking about ourselves and our circumstances – that is what we are referring to, for example, when we describe somebody as an optimist or a pessimist. These habitual ways of thinking are important because they influence how we react to circumstances, sometimes leading us to make false assumptions about the meaning of what is happening or what we can do about it – assuming, for example, that what someone has said is more critical or blaming than it was meant to be, or that there's nothing we can do about some new problem.

This idea has attracted much attention recently because thoughts, sometimes referred to by the technical word *cognitions,* are the focus of a therapy you may have heard of called cognitive or cognitive behavioural therapy (CBT). The idea of CBT is to identify these ways of thinking and to challenge them so that the person can try to change the way they think and therefore how they behave towards themselves and others. There is more about CBT later in this book.

One example of a style of thinking that may lead to self-harm is a tendency to *hopeless thinking* about the future: that is, an automatically pessimistic or negative response to events, with an assumption that things will always turn out badly. This way of thinking usually comes from a combination of experiences that leads to a sense of powerlessness – typically, encountering unpleasant events and being unable to influence what effect those experiences have. Not surprisingly then, when something new and challenging happens, a person with these earlier experiences assumes the worst.

Another thinking style that can be easy to identify is *black and white thinking* – a way of viewing the world that deals in definite 'either–or' portrayals, and which miss out the possibility of 'in-between' or grey areas. For example, 'If everything isn't OK it's a disaster.'

We'd been going out for about four months when he told me he wanted to finish our relationship. I was gutted. I don't find it easy being close to people and he just seemed right for me. I thought … this is it, this is my life … I'll always be on my own.

Joanne, 18

These ways of thinking and responding to circumstances can have the effect of limiting someone's flexibility when it comes to dealing with stressful events or circumstances.

Most of us, when faced with distressing circumstances in life, respond in one of two main ways. We do what is called emotional coping – finding ways to manage the anxiety, sadness or anger that comes as a natural response to what has happened: crying on a friend's shoulder or going to the gym for a hard workout to take our mind off it for a while. And we also try *practical coping* – finding things to do that reduce the impact of what has happened: drawing up a plan of action. If a person's habitual attitude is that the outcome of such action plans is likely to be negative, or if they think in extremes, then it is difficult for them to adopt the approach 'suppose I try such-and-such, maybe that will help a little'. And indeed, many people who self-harm have difficulty with problem-solving.

When I got a letter from the bank saying they were foreclosing on my business, I didn't know what to do. I thought of all the people I owed money, all the customers I had let down, how badly it would affect my family. I phoned the bank but they were adamant they wouldn't extend my loan. I just couldn't think what else to do – it just seemed like the end of the road.

Dan, 48

Some of these ways of thinking can be challenged and changed as a part of therapy: see Chapter 8 for more on this.

Self-harm and other damaging actions

We have already noted that people who self-harm may also engage in other self-damaging actions such as drinking recklessly or following an abnormal eating pattern. One well-known finding from research is that self-harm is also associated with aggression. Why should that be? Actually, when you think about it, it isn't surprising – all acts of self-harm are a sort of attack on the body so maybe the question is not, 'Why is self-harm associated with aggression?' but 'Why is aggression sometimes directed towards the self and sometimes towards other people?' One reason is that self-harm could act as substitution for hurting others.

I first started harming myself at school. Some of the other lads were teasing me about my mum and especially this lad Andy was winding me up. I could feel the anger building up inside me and it was so strong I was frightened what I might do to him if I started on him. When I harmed myself it seemed to let something out of me somehow.

Geoff, 34

We will return to this question in the next chapter about reasons for self-harm, when we talk about the need for self-punishment. For now, it is just worth noting again how often self-harm hangs out with other self-destructive actions such as misuse of drugs and alcohol.

Psychiatric disorders and self-harm

The commonest mental disorder that leads to self-harm is severe depression. That's because depression as an illness can cause a state of intolerable suffering, and also because it can bring on feelings of hopelessness, even if that hopeless way of thinking isn't the individual's usual style.

There is a group of psychiatric disorders like schizophrenia and bipolar illness that are sometimes called the 'severe mental illnesses'. Their symptoms are sometimes called psychotic because when the illness is at its worst, the person may hear frightening or compelling voices telling them what to do or abusing them, or they might have abnormal beliefs (called delusions) that cannot be shifted by logic or argument.

In an acute hospital, it turns out that very few people who come for help (physical or mental) after self-harm are affected with schizophrenia or bipolar illness. When you do see those people seeking help for self-harm, sometimes the psychotic symptoms themselves (such as hearing voices or holding abnormal beliefs) explain their self-harm. However, at other times their self-harming is associated with social problems – unemployment, poverty, social isolation. In those cases it is not the psychosis but the social difficulties that lead to the self-harm.

Although it is widely assumed that hearing voices is always a symptom of psychosis, it is not that uncommon for people to hear voices when they have no other experiences or symptoms to suggest psychosis. In this situation, hearing voices is still important and distressing and can indeed be associated with self-harm. If this is your experience, don't be too frightened to tell someone; that is, don't assume that they will take it as a sign of madness. A mental health professional should be able to discuss with you what it is about and what you might do about it.

It is worth mentioning anorexia nervosa at this point. Its severest form is not common, but milder types of eating disorder, which are common in young women, are also linked to self-harm. The most likely explanation is that dislike of the body and its weight and shape is almost invariably part of a wider self-dislike. If such self-dislike is expressed in one bodily way (through disordered eating) then it would be consistent to see another bodily expression of emotion (self-harm) in the same person. It is also true that both self-harm and eating disorders are ways of taking control in circumstances that otherwise feel impossible to manage.

For a sense of perspective, here's a picture of the hospital self-harm service that I worked in. We asked the self-harm team to make a record of psychiatric disorders in 1,000 people who they saw. This is what they found:

Psychotic disorders	5%
Severe mood disorder (including bipolar)	5%
Mild/moderate depression	10%
Alcohol and substance misuse	10%
Other disorders (including anorexia, OCD, autism, etc.)	5%
No psychiatric disorder	65%

In other words, although everybody they saw had

troubles and was distressed at the time they were seen, psychiatric diagnosis wasn't an especially good way of describing what the problem was for the majority. And looking at it the other way round gives a rather similar picture – although self-harm is common in people with a diagnosis of mental illness, it is reported only in a minority. For example, a recent study of people having their first episode of psychotic illness found that only about one in ten had self-harmed as part of this first illness. The message is that psychiatric illness and self-harm are associated, but that diagnosing mental illness isn't a good way of explaining self-harm in most cases.

Lastly in this section, let's look at learning disability. It's true that learning disability isn't a psychiatric disorder, it is (as its name suggests) a disability rather than a disorder, but lots of people with a learning disability do have mental health problems. Recent surveys have found that rates of self-harm are high in adults with a learning disability. This has been called 'challenging behaviour', as if it's somehow a behavioural problem caused by having a learning disability, but in fact the causes of self-harm – such as worry about physical illness or bullying or loneliness – are probably the same as they are for other adults. All that's different is that it's harder, if you have a learning disability, to know how to get help for your problems because of not knowing how to ask for it.

Personality and self-harm

To my mind, one of the most unhelpful ways that psychiatry has of talking about people and their problems is the use of diagnostic labels to describe somebody's personality. Psychiatrists talk about *personality disorder* to label the situation when certain ways of thinking, feeling or behaving are persistent in someone over many years and are harmful to that individual or to others around them.

There are real problems with this way of thinking. First, and rather obviously, it leads to an emphasis on the individual as the source of their problems and therefore downplays the role of other people and circumstances.

Dorothy, a trainee nurse, lived with her unemployed and controlling partner in a flat where they had fallen into rent arrears. His behaviour meant that she missed work and he mocked her studying so she had to do it secretly. Her performance dropped and her supervisor discussed letting her go. One night the police were called. She was threatening her partner with a hammer, which she then threw out through the first-floor window. At the police station, the duty doctor found that she had multiple scars from self-harm on her thighs. She was diagnosed with a personality disorder and told there was no cure for it.

In this situation it is clear that the diagnostic label,

which described the problems as being as a result of her personal psychology, obscured the real social and personal dilemmas with which Dorothy was struggling and made the search for solutions more difficult.

Second, the diagnosis is often experienced as a way of saying 'the problem is about who you are as a person' and it is widely used in a critical or dismissive way by professionals in health and social care. The person on the receiving end can easily be stigmatised and become (rightly) angry – that anger then being used as further evidence of what's wrong with them. Not surprisingly, lots of people given this diagnosis don't like it and don't like the effect it has on the way others treat them.

This isn't to say that people don't have recognisable and enduring characteristics. We all know somebody who is particularly obsessional, prickly, paranoid or prone to emotional outbursts. Sometimes these characteristics do indeed seem important in explaining self-harm. For example, impulsivity is a tendency to act on the spur of the moment, without much thought and without consideration of the consequences. This characteristic is quite commonly associated with self-harm, especially when it is coupled with negative ways of thinking.

I spoke with Andy during his hospital admission on a trauma ward. He had stepped in front of a lorry and had survived with broken bones but no life-threatening injury. He told me:

I was standing on the pavement thinking about what had gone wrong in my life and I was feeling pretty bad about it all. I'd planned to see my girlfriend that evening but I was thinking – what's the point, it's not going anywhere? This truck came round the corner and I just thought that second – go for it – and I stepped out. When I think about it now I don't want to die but just at that moment I didn't care.

What isn't right is elevating these observations into diagnostic statements – putting people into categories as if somebody's personality is a mental disorder – which is indeed where personality disorder sits in the main diagnostic systems used worldwide.

There's another practical problem with this 'diagnostic' approach to personality, which is how little use it is in explaining anything.

A fellow psychiatrist told me about an encounter in her student years:

Medical student: Why has Ms Smith taken an overdose?

Psychiatrist: Well, she's had an argument and broken up with her partner, but the main reason is that she has a personality disorder.

Medical student: Is that a medical diagnosis?

Psychiatrist: Yes, she has an emotionally unstable or borderline personality disorder.

Medical student: How did you diagnose that?

Psychiatrist: Her relationships don't last, she is emotionally unpredictable and she presents frequently after episodes of self-harm.

The student left it at that, but was acutely aware of the circular diagnosis as 'explanation'. This circular reasoning is really common in practice; in other words, using repeated self-harm as part of the basis for diagnosing a personality disorder and then using the diagnosed 'condition' to explain the repeated self-harm.

It is important to say that many mental health professionals do not share my doubts about the value of a diagnosis of personality disorder. Also, while many patients object to being labelled in this way there are some who value the diagnosis, either because it helps them think about their problems, making them more manageable, or because having a diagnosis gives them a right of access to mental health services. In the light of this, it is important to be clear about what may be meant when the term is used by those professionals who find it useful.

In broad terms, psychiatrists now talk about personality disorders as falling into three groups or clusters:

◆ prickly, paranoid or withdrawn personality disorders
◆ antisocial – often called psychopathic or sociopathic personality disorder
◆ emotionally unstable – including borderline personality disorder.

It is the third type especially that has come to be linked to self-harm. The main basis for the diagnosis is the presence of four features:

◆ emotional instability
◆ disturbed patterns of thinking or perception

◆ impulsive behaviour – including episodes of self-harm
◆ intense but unstable relationships with others.

Whatever you think about diagnosing personality, pretty much everybody who works in trying to help people who self-harm will agree about where to start: the best care and support involves helping the person to find new ways of responding to stress, regardless of their diagnosis. We will also return to therapy for self-harm in Chapter 8, when I talk about seeking help from mental health services.

Having talked about personal characteristics, we can now say something about how such characteristics develop. Are we all just born a certain way? If so, does that mean that we can't do anything about how we respond to stress? Or are there other influences that we can learn to understand and then modify in terms of their effect on us?

Origins of personal characteristics linked to self-harm

Is genetics important?

It's quite common to hear parents say of their grown-up children that they had certain stand-out characteristics from a very early age, for example that they were prone to prefer their own company, or get easily upset, or worry incessantly about something that seemed trivial to an adult. And we meet people who seem to have grown up to be just like one of their parents. This raises the question of how much of who we are is hereditary, or in our genes.

It isn't easy to answer this question. The research that tries to do so typically takes one of two forms. In classical genetic studies researchers have studied family trees, asking, for example, if identical twins are more like each other than non-identical twins or non-twin brothers and sisters. In modern research, blood tests can study the human genes or the molecules they code for. This research is still in its infancy but it has provided us with some pointers.

Certainly, there is a genetic cause to some mental illnesses, such as bipolar disorder. Most learning disability has genetic causes. It also seems that certain psychological characteristics are influenced at least in part by genes. However, the genetic link to personality is not that clear-cut – lots of genes seem to have an influence on aspects of behaviour but there isn't a strong, simple link in the way that there is for some hereditary diseases. And genetics can't explain the way self-harm rates vary over quite short periods of time and in different parts of the country – there must be other reasons at play.

Early life experiences

It has long been understood that early life experiences are influential in shaping the sort of person we grow up to be. The most important influences explored in this book are those through which we learn how to form and maintain relationships, and those that affect how we come to think of ourselves in later life.

There are some important early physical influences on how we develop – inadequate nutrition is relatively uncommon in the developed world, but serious childhood illness and disability is still not that rare. Nearly 4 per cent of school-age children are noted on the National Pupil Database in the UK as having some special educational need, much of it related to physical illness or chronic disability (including learning disability).

However, the biggest influence on personal, emotional and psychological development is the relationship we have with parents or other significant adults in our early lives. There are times when self-harm by young people appears to come out of the blue but research shows that a depressingly large proportion of adults who have harmed themselves have a story of unhappy early life experiences.

Professionals who work with children distinguish between *neglectful* upbringings, where something is missing that should be provided for a child or young person during their early life, and *abusive* upbringings, where a child or young person is exposed to actively unpleasant, wrong or damaging experiences rather than just being deprived of desirable experiences. In each case – neglect or abuse – the experiences may be emotional, physical or sexual.

My dad used to be really party-loving and outgoing, but when he'd had a drink we saw the other side of him. He'd knock my mum around and if my older brother tried to protect her he'd hit him too. He started hitting me when

I was 13. Once he hit me so hard I had bruises all over my arms and I stayed off school until they were gone; I was too scared to tell anybody what happened because I knew he'd hit me again if I did. I used to be angry with him, and with mum for not leaving him and protecting us. He used to say it was our fault for winding him up and I suppose I did always blame myself in some way – felt I wasn't worth anything better.

Josie, 23

Most attention is given, both by professionals and in the media, to physical or sexual abuse. Both are particularly damaging when they occur in the family – when the young person is a victim of domestic violence or when the perpetrator of sexual abuse is a family member or close family friend. The reason is, at least in part, that the betrayal of trust leads to difficulty in forming trusting and intimate relationships in later life. Also, survivors of abuse often blame themselves for what happened and so grow up with a low sense of self-worth.

This last point brings us to the hugely important topic of emotional abuse and emotional neglect. Until recently these experiences have received less attention than physical or sexual abuse because they are hard to demonstrate to others, since they leave no physical evidence, but they are often behind stories from people in distress.

When he was at home, it was like me dad were the only important thing to me mam – what he wanted ... keeping

*him happy. We had to be quiet when he wanted to watch
telly, play with him when he wanted to play with us. We
did everything to please him and when he were happy we
were happy. But when I look back now I can see – it were
all about him. He weren't interested in us for us own sakes
– just because we were 'his' children. He never cuddled us
when we cried or owt like that. I can see that, now I've had
me own children.*

Beth, 52

Increasingly we have come to understand this point:
that emotional abuse and neglect can be as damaging
as the more obvious forms of physical and sexual abuse
in the effect they have on our sense of self-esteem, our
well-being and our ability to form trusting relationships
in later life.

Later life experiences

Although we tend to think of early life experiences,
especially up to puberty, as being important in determining who we are, there are also important later
influences. New relationships are important emotionally and practically.

One of the great difficulties for those who have
grown up in troubled circumstances is how hard it is
for them to trust other people. They either keep their
distance, or they fall quickly into relationships that then
don't last.

*I hate being on my own. I spent all my childhood like that
– no friends at school, nobody I talked to on my street. I*

hung out with a gang of lads for a while but they were
always getting into trouble and they only wanted me
around because I was a big lad not because they liked me.
I lived with Carol for eighteen months but I messed it up –
always thought she was going with somebody else, used to
resent her having friends, so in the end she got fed up and
left me.

Martin, 32

This sort of uncertain way of relating to other people has practical consequences as well as emotional ones. As mentioned earlier, people who self-harm often have poor problem-solving skills: one of the resources we use when solving problems is other people's ideas, and how can we do that if we don't trust the people closest to us or we avoid developing intimate relationships?

A word of comfort to parents. Many parents discovering for the first time that their child has harmed themselves immediately wonder what they did wrong, and how they can make it right.

I could not believe it when I discovered that Charlotte
had been taken to hospital with an overdose, and I nearly
collapsed when it turned out that this was not the first time.
How could I not have known? What did I do to create this
situation? Her mother and I had a stand-up row outside
the hospital about how we had missed it, and whose fault it
was, and then we just cried all night.

Malcolm, Charlotte's father

There's no need to get caught up in self-blame about what has happened. Most of us do the best we can in bringing up our children. Often we have considerable challenges of our own, just living the best life we can. If your child has self-harmed, now is not the time to agonise over what has caused your particular family crisis. It is time to focus on making things better. It won't be easy. And there may be times when you have to stand back and allow others to do this work.

At the hospital they invited families to the case conferences, but our daughter refused to consent to us taking part. She wouldn't even let us visit. We had to let it go. She was over 18 already then.

Malcolm, Charlotte's father

Taking stock: what we know about the background to acts of self-harm

If you ask somebody who has recently self-harmed about the reason for it, one common response is for them to give a description of stressful circumstances or experiences. It could be the break-up of an important relationship, mounting debt, or tension or arguments at home. You can see lots of examples of this on the websites of those organisations that support people seeking help for mental health problems and self-harm.

We had started a business that was meant to be a fantastic success. It had everything going for it, but we just needed some more cash ... and then my partner just walked out at the same time as the bank was pressing me. I couldn't sleep for worry. I was in a constant state of panic. It was all my fault. I just took the tablets and later when I felt sick

I panicked even more and wished I hadn't done it – that's why I came to the hospital.

Austin, 32

They bully me at school because I always get high grades. They call me 'academy snob'. I tried to do less, to drop grades, but then I got into trouble at home and the teachers were always on to me. The first time I scratched myself with the metal tab off a soda can. Then I started with razor blades from the art classroom.

Fiona, 17

Of course, many people have stress like this in their lives but for some reason they don't respond by harming themselves.

The next question that Fiona or Austin might be asked could be something like – 'Yes, I can see that's stressful. But what was it that made you self-harm when it happened to you? Why did it seem the right course of action at the time?'

We've already looked at certain personal charac-teristics that make it more likely that somebody will self-harm. This may be particular ways that they have of thinking about their problems. It could be a per-sonal style, such as a tendency to be aggressive or to act impulsively. They may have mental health problems or they may be thought to have persistent aspects to their personality that make certain actions more likely.

It is important to remember that these elements are not the whole story for self-harm. The fact that someone's individual way of thinking or their usual behaviour is a factor in explaining self-harm does not mean that their distressing situation or circumstances are irrelevant. It can be too easy to put someone's self-harm down to a problem with their personality. What they are living through might be difficult or even nightmarish for any person.

The message of hope from this is that people who self-harm may be able to learn, or teach themselves, how other people deal with horrible situations or feelings, and that just getting out of the bad situation in itself can make a huge difference. It may even allow them to stop, or to imagine a time when they will be able to.

A recent research study asked how people with a history of repeated self-harm managed to stop. The results showed that we can all change dramatically when circumstances change dramatically: three significant reasons given for how young people were able to stop self-harming were that they left an abusive home environment; started a supportive relationship; or stopped drinking.

In the following chapters, I want to look at the challenge of explaining self-harm in a different way. When trying to understand somebody's self-harm, I may recognise that they have had certain stressful experiences, and it may be that I identify personal characteristics that increase the chances that they will self-harm. But that still does not fully indicate *why* this person has decided to take this action. What are the *reasons* for self-harm? What function was it meant to serve? That's what the next chapters are about.

chapter 3

Self-harm and attempted suicide

This chapter will discuss the really important question of the relationship between self-harm and attempted suicide. We have already seen how some acts of self-harm are attempts at suicide, but many are not. This chapter explores whether we can identify those acts of self-harm that are failed attempts at suicide, or are warnings that suicide is imminent. Can we tell them apart from those acts that were never intended to be fatal? It is obvious why this is important. If you can tell who is most likely to kill themselves, you may be able to save a life.

Non-fatal self-harm and attempted suicide

The way in which things are described, and the language we use, is important. It can reveal your attitude to what somebody does or even the way you feel about the person themselves, and therefore influence how easy it is to have a discussion about suicidal thoughts and suicide risk.

When a family member, or a health or social worker, is trying to work out what is going on, the words that are used in public discussions can influence their response. People have in the past been described by hospitals as 'time-wasters' because they did something that didn't look like a serious attempt at suicide, and yet still came to hospital for medical treatment. People talk about 'committing' suicide as if it is a crime, which it is not. There is a tendency among coroners to avoid judging that a death was by suicide because of religious stigma, or even for insurance considerations. The correct use of technical language is important, whether it is in reporting or in general discussion.

When an experienced professional in this field labels any act of self-harm as attempted suicide, they are saying that in their judgement the desired aim was to end life, either immediately or in the near future. They are evaluating the person's intention. Only if they believed self-harm was part of a build-up to a final act would they describe it as suicidal. This desire to die is sometimes called *suicidal intent*.

Let me say a couple of things straight away. The first is that it is difficult, even for professionals, to decide whether there really is suicidal intent. You sometimes hear health professionals talk about 'risk assessment', which usually means that a sort of checklist will be used to make predictions about what will happen next. Typically, the list will include answers to questions such as self-reported intentions, and the health professional will note psychiatric symptoms and the immediate circumstances of the act of self-harm. The problem with this approach is that it just isn't an accurate way to predict the future.

Psychiatrists often want to know if there's a useful way to measure suicide risk after a non-fatal act of self-harm. The truth is that there isn't. Prediction of suicide is so inaccurate that we don't advise the routine use of any risk scales. That isn't to say that psychiatrists shouldn't ask questions about intent, it's just that they must be realistic about how accurate risk assessment is in predicting what happens next. By far the best course of action is to make a careful assessment of somebody's needs and develop a plan with them about what to do next.

Dr Nav Kapur, professor of psychiatry

The second thing to say is that friends and family, who will inevitably feel worried, should not feel that they have to make a judgement about suicide risk. If somebody close to you harms themselves you should seek help from a professional who should be able to both offer your friend or family help and to advise you about what you can do.

Research shows that the risk of suicide after self-harm is indeed high. The suicide rate in people who have been seen at a hospital after self-harm is about 50 times greater than it is in the general population.

Why is it so difficult to judge whether somebody is at risk of suicide even after an act of self-harm? Although you can always ask someone what they intended you might be afraid that they won't tell you the truth, perhaps because they want to conceal their plans from you in case you stop them. Many people are afraid to ask someone if they intend to kill themselves, as if the very act of asking might put the idea into their mind. We may wonder if talking about it makes suicide seem more comprehensible, if not acceptable, and may nudge the person in that direction. You should not think like this – there is no evidence that asking people about suicide will put it into their mind when they weren't already thinking about it, and therefore make them more likely to kill themselves. In fact, *not* asking people how they are feeling is more likely to send an unintended message that there are things you don't want to know about.

So, is it just a question of asking people about their intentions? One problem is that if we ask people, they are often vague or unclear about their motives at the time, especially if they'd been drinking. Or they have mixed feelings, or what they think now isn't what they felt at the time. It also depends on who is asking and what the circumstances are.

My mother asked me why I did it and I wasn't going to say to her face, 'It was to get away from you.'

Eleanor, 16

My dad thinks you go into eternal damnation and hell if you kill yourself, so I just said that I'd drunk the weed killer by accident from a whisky bottle. I don't mind telling you, though, I'm sorry I'm alive. I don't want to spend another winter on that farm. I'm so lonely and tired.

Fraser, 36

I don't know what I was thinking. I was just stupid drunk and fell out with my mates.

Margaret, 24

And it's very common that the response you get to a question about motive is, 'I just wanted out of it all – to switch off from all my problems.' What is described frequently sounds like a sort of search for oblivion, so in one way it's quite worrying, but in another way it's saying, 'No, I wasn't trying to kill myself.'

Another important factor that makes prediction difficult is that suicide after self-harm is quite rare. That seems odd when I have just said that it is relatively common – about 50 times as common as suicide in the general population. The important word is 'relatively'. Here's the explanation.

The suicide rate in the general population is about one per year for every 10,000 people. Suppose I live in a small town of 10,000 people. Statistically, you might expect one of my fellow inhabitants to kill themselves in any year. Now, to build the risk caused by self-harm into the picture, imagine the nearest big city with two million residents – there will be quite a lot of people in that city who harm themselves in any one year. Maybe they've been seen at a clinic, or the hospital, or in the GP surgery, or they are being quiet at home. Let's say there are 10,000 people in that city who see a health professional each year after an episode of self-harm. If suicide is only as common in this group as in the general population then I'd expect one of these people to die by suicide in the next year. But we know that suicide is at least 50 times more frequent in this group – so, I'd expect 50 of them to kill themselves in the next year. This means that 9,950 of the 10,000 people who self-harm do *not* kill themselves in the next year. So, suicide is still quite uncommon. One person dead from suicide is too many, but identifying 50 with suicidal intention among 10,000 people who self-harm is quite difficult, so much so that it is impossible to spot every one. That's why I can say that suicide after self-harm is quite rare: it is hard to sift through everyone and find the lost ones before it is too late. Fortunately, we can say that this problem of difficulty in prediction is caused by the fact that most people don't kill themselves.

Suicidal intent, then, is difficult to judge because people can't always tell you themselves, and suicide is difficult to predict because it's not a common outcome in the months after self-harm. Finally, suicide is difficult to predict because circumstances change. Just because a particular act wasn't accompanied by strong suicidal ideas doesn't mean that the person involved is at no risk of suicide. It depends what happens next in their story.

He never talked about suicide and when I asked him he said he wouldn't do it. But I suppose looking back now I should have seen that he always had it in him – after I knew he'd harmed himself before I mean ... I suppose I think ... he can't have cared that much about himself to do that, can he? So, when he got depressed again (after Josie left) he just turned it in on himself.

John, 38, talking about his friend's suicide

I need to say something here about what is called *non-suicidal self-injury*, which has been defined as 'the intentional destruction of one's own body tissue without suicidal intent and for purposes not socially sanctioned'. This is an idea strongly favoured by clinicians and researchers, especially in the US. It is less popular in the UK for the reasons I have touched on about how difficult it can be for people to be clear about their intentions. From my point of view the most important consideration is that I am interested in suicidal intent as it applies to an individual rather than to an act of self-harm. Of course it's clear that some self-harm is not driven by suicidal thoughts, and that some people will repeatedly harm themselves and say that they don't intend to die, but I think it is unwise to accept that certain types of self-harm (especially cutting) are 'non-suicidal'. And the fact that somebody says that their self-harm is not suicidal cannot be taken as reassurance that they will not become suicidal later and take their own life.

All of which isn't to say that health professionals take no notice of ideas about suicide risk – they consider it all the time. But it may be more accurate to say that they use particular signs to alert them to take extra special care about offering the right help to certain people.

When I see somebody for assessment after self-harm, certain factors ring the alarm bells for me:

- *if the person is older than the average, especially if they are male,*

- *if they have done something unusual or especially violent like attempted hanging, or planned it carefully and made special attempts not to be discovered,*

- *if their reasons suggest real hopelessness or they have*

other symptoms like severe depression,

– *if they have a history of psychiatric treatment for mental illness.*

All these factors are commoner in people who die by suicide so I take special notice then. I don't like the idea of turning them into a score like some people do, but you just feel they are worth taking note of when you are treating somebody.

Psychiatric nurse working in an emergency department

I'll finish this section by repeating something I said earlier. Of course suicide risk is a worry and should always be taken seriously. But if you know somebody socially or in your family who has self-harmed it is not your job to assess suicide risk. It is vital that you ask for professional help. And if you are somebody who self-harms yourself and you want help, don't accept it if you are told that you can't have help because somebody has done a risk assessment and says you are at low risk. As NICE says, the help you are offered should be based on your needs and not on someone's 'risk assessment'.

In the next chapters I will look at other reasons for self-harm, and discuss the apparently unusual idea that self-harm isn't just a symptom but that it can serve a purpose.

chapter 4

Self-harm as a way of responding to distress

It is generally true, and some people assert that it absolutely goes without saying, that when somebody self-harms they are distressed or troubled. You will, however, sometimes hear dismissive comments about self-harm like, 'She's only doing it for attention', or 'He just wants to use it as an excuse to get out of trouble.' Even if (and it's a big if) these observations have some truth to them, you might still ask: 'Yes, that's possible, but how troubled does somebody have to be if they are prepared to harm themselves for attention or to avoid another difficulty? And how odd is it to think that this is a good way of getting attention?' I am persuaded that even if somebody's actions *seem* to be manipulative (seeking attention), the fact that they use this extraordinary method is certainly a sign of being troubled.

Sometimes people say that self-harm is a 'symptom' or a 'sign' of distress. In healthcare, we often talk about signs and symptoms of problems. A sign of diabetes might be a raised blood sugar level in a blood test. Symptoms might include being thirsty and tired. The difference is that a sign is something that someone else can measure, but the thirst and the tiredness have to be experienced in order to know that they are happening. That personal experience is what is called a symptom.

Self-harm is a sign of distress, and if you ask carefully you can nearly always find the symptoms of that distress, but there is more to it than that. This chapter will consider the idea that self-harm isn't in this sense just a *sign* of distress. Rather, it is also the person's way of *dealing with* distress.

To explain why that might be, we will explore the idea that self-harm serves a purpose for the person doing it. It has one or more *functions*, aside from being a symptom. This is a complex idea and these various functions can't be ranked in order of importance, but we have to start somewhere. Some of the reasons for self-harm outlined in this chapter and the next really apply only to someone who harms themselves repeatedly; and some of the information here applies especially to somebody who has harmed themselves just once, for example by taking an overdose in the middle of a personal crisis. So don't be surprised if everything here doesn't apply to you or to someone close to you; there's nothing that can sensibly be applied to everybody who self-harms. Everyone is different.

Let's start with the premise that one of the functions of self-harm may be to allow the person to cope with distress – not an ideal way of coping, but it is their way.

One indication that this idea may be valid is that sometimes the method of self-harm is obviously related to the reason for it, and certain methods are associated with particular reasons. For example, if you want to inflict pain on yourself as a punishment then you are more likely to cut or burn yourself rather than to take an overdose of tablets. But remember that people have a mixture of reasons for self-harm, and these can vary over time. It can be difficult for the outside observer to see a pattern.

There's another reason why it can be difficult to judge what the motives are for self-harm. Some people can find it easy to explain why they self-harmed while others find it difficult to think about why it happened and what they did to themselves. Any one person's reasons for self-harm can be easy for them to describe or they can be difficult for them to pin down or to find the words for. Here is an example of someone who has a well worked-out reason on each of two separate occasions.

I have hurt myself twice this week. On Monday I just knew all day that I wanted to – I had a bad weekend feeling low and drinking on my own in my flat. I went to work with a hangover and just hated myself for being such a loser. When I'm like that I know that cutting myself lets it out of me somehow and I felt a bit better. As always, I promised myself I wouldn't do it again. On Thursday, my boss saw I had a bandage on the forearm and made a joke about it, something like 'Ooh, you haven't been cutting your wrist, have you?' He is completely insensitive and he won't have thought that was what it was but it made me angry that he thought cutting yourself is funny. I thought – it's nothing to do with you what I do, it's up to me and it's my body – and

*I did it again as a sort of way of saying that to myself, and
I suppose of getting the anger out of my system.*

Louise, 22

Others are not so clear.

*It's a thing I do when I am drunk. I'm not the only one,
am I? It's something people do when they're fed up. I've got
mates who do it.*

Fred, 28

Controlling emotions

It is well known that doing something physical can make
you feel better emotionally. Going for a run or a swim
or a workout at the gym can be a distraction and it can
lift depressed feelings even if only temporarily. There
are other ways of using our physical bodies to improve
our mental state. The effects of alcohol or recreational
drugs, when used in a certain way, include a calming
effect on anxiety and tension, which accounts in part
for their popularity. Of course, these things don't work
for everybody but it is an everyday observation that the
state of our bodies affects our emotions in the same
way that our emotions affect how we feel physically.

Not surprisingly, therefore, a physical act like self-
harm can have the same effect. Academics sometimes
call this process 'emotional regulation' (meaning 'managing feelings') or you may come across the term *affect
regulation*, which means the same thing. There seem to be
different ways in which self-harm helps control feelings.

One way that self-harm may improve emotional states is by the power of expectation: you feel better after self-harm because you expect to. I am struck by how often people overdose with drugs designed to kill pain – physical painkillers like paracetamol, or emotional painkillers like tranquillisers. Another significant aspect of the story is how often somebody lies down or goes to bed after an overdose, even if they haven't taken a sedating drug. It says to me that what they are seeking is calm, rest, escape from emotional pain and turmoil.

Many of the tablets taken in overdose have mood-altering effects, typically with a sedative action.

It doesn't matter what I do to harm myself … if I take tablets I use strong painkillers and it just seems to numb the emotional pain for a while. If I cut myself I find the physical pain is easier to bear than the emotional pain, perhaps it's easier to understand so I know how to be strong enough to deal with it.

Asma, 25

And, as Asma told me, the physical pain caused by self-injury can be powerful enough in itself and can have a meaning that is comforting.

One particularly unpleasant emotional state is a sense of unreality – a feeling of being disconnected from the world or from one's own body. It's difficult to describe, but I find that anyone who has experienced this state understands straight away what I am talking about. It is technically known as *depersonalisation* or *derealisation*.

Sometimes I get this horrible empty feeling like I'm not there – I look in the mirror and it's as if I'm looking at a stranger I don't know … just no feeling, but there is a feeling that's dreadful, I can't describe. It usually passes but once, when it was lasting, I burned myself with a match and the pain seemed to bring me back to life somehow.

Marie, 43

The main problem with using self-harm to control emotions is that even if it works in the short term (and it doesn't always) the bad feelings come back after a while – now with the added burden of thoughts about the episode of self-harm.

Self-punishment

As a psychiatrist I meet lots of people who have had troubled, unhappy or deprived lives. It always saddens me when they say that they blame themselves for what has happened to them, as if they deserve the way they have been treated. Sometimes this happens because abusive people are good at blaming their victims and the victim may internalise this guilt. That's why people who have recovered don't like even being called 'victim' and prefer the term 'survivor', if they are to be labelled at all.

At times it seems to be a way that some people respond to the world, assuming that what happens to them must have been brought on by who they are. Punishing yourself is then like a way of seeking forgiveness.

Harming myself is a way of proving to myself how worthless I am, what a bad person. It's like a way of punishing myself for who I am. When I do it I think … you deserve this.

Andy, 19

I have to cut myself deeply enough to make it bleed. It's as if the blood releases something … it's a strange feeling … like it washes away all the badness from inside me.

Anju, 22

Switching off thoughts and memories

Distress isn't just an emotional state – it comes with negative thoughts about yourself or about other people or about what might happen in the future. And it comes with memories, usually bad memories that can intrude even when you don't want them. Self-harm, because it is so powerful an experience in the here and now, can be a way of distancing or blocking those thoughts and memories.

It's like a torture, these thoughts just going round and round in my head. Maybe about something small like what somebody at work has said to me or maybe something big and vague like what I'm going to do with my life. I can't stop them … but if I've taken some tablets then when they kick in I notice it all just matters less and then it seems like the thoughts drift off and I just notice how floaty I feel. Of course, it's all back when I come to.

Charlie, 36

When I'm on my own, especially at night, the memories come to me of what he did. Especially the last time … it was just so horrible, I relive every second of it. The only way I can get rid of it is to hurt myself – the pain takes my mind off it and then there's all the faff of cleaning up afterwards, putting on a bandage, trying to find a way to hide it from other people.

Emily, 24

I think sometimes about him and how much he hurt me … betrayed me really and let me down. I'd trusted him and he knew that. So when I do something it's like he's there and … I don't know. Am I thinking 'look what you made me do?' … or is it like 'You're nothing, you didn't hurt me as much as I can hurt myself.' Whatever … it seems to push him out of my mind.

Alexe, 42

Communicating distress to others

For many people self-harm is a deeply personal and private act; perhaps embarrassing or shameful, perhaps something that defines who they are and that isn't anybody else's business. If they have scars they hide them from others. They only tell somebody when they need direct help, for example with the medical complications of what they have done.

When I got home I was just so angry and upset … and I suppose I was a bit drunk because we'd spent the night in the pub. I paced around in my room and just got more and more wound up and in the end I went to the bathroom and took the tablets. Pretty much straight away I regretted it and so I went to bed and thought – I'll sleep it off and nobody will know. Then I woke in the night and felt awful; I was sick. I got frightened that I'd done myself damage so I woke my mum and she took me to the hospital.

Angelina, 17

However, some people are able to disclose their self-harm – maybe as a way of seeking help in less direct ways than in the example above.

There's a boy who stops and talks to me sometimes when I am helping in the shop. He is just being friendly but my brother told our father that I was seen with him in town and that he was bringing shame on our family. My father got angry. I tried to tell him that in this country [the family is from West Africa] it is OK for boys to talk to girls like this but he wouldn't listen and he dragged me around the room shouting about how I had disgraced him, and he hit me so I was bruised and had to stay off school. I was so sad … I felt like I didn't want to go on and I took some tablets. After, I told my mum but she just got angry. I think I did it partly because I wanted her to listen, to understand me and to talk to my dad.

Patience, 18

Letting other people know about self-harm isn't only about seeking help or support. Simply sharing can bring relief – at least somebody else knows what I'm struggling with. Sometimes an entirely different sort of response is what's wanted.

I asked Jacqui why she wore a short-sleeved T-shirt: her scars are very prominent and it provokes stares. She told me, *'I want them to know I don't do nothing to please others.'* When I explored further she told me she liked the way her scars upset and yet fascinated other people. It made her feel … *'I dunno, like if it upsets you then good, this is what my life's like. This is who I am. I'm strong enough to take it well, I am.'*

Warding off suicide

As we have seen, people who self harm have a much higher rate of suicide than others. Much more common than actual suicide is having thoughts about suicide – imagining it, thinking about what it would be like and how it would affect others, wondering what you'd do, perhaps even making plans. If these thoughts are more frequent than actual suicide, it suggests that people are able to overcome them with some effort. Surprisingly, self-harm seems to be one of the things that helps people who feel suicidal to stave off actually acting on their feelings.

Sometimes I hear my dad in my head, telling me I'm a waste of space and I'll never make anything of myself. And I can think – he was right, everything I do is a failure. I'll never do any better, why don't I just end it now? Harming myself feels like a way of meeting those thoughts halfway – I can't defeat them altogether but it's like I put a full stop to them.

Jim, 27, outpatient clinic

It's important to be clear about this. You can't assume that somebody who thinks about suicide is not going to kill themselves simply because their self-harm protects them. Sometimes the exact opposite is true.

My self-harm feels like a sort of practice ... getting used to the idea of killing myself. It's a bit like if I kill a little bit of myself now, I can be ready to do the whole job when I decide to.

Maria, 48

Luckily, this way of thinking isn't common. So, the message is – don't panic. Help is available, and sometimes, although discovering that somebody is self-harming is disturbing, it's worth remembering that it may be their way of coping with their distress. And remember: if you are a friend or relative of somebody who harms themselves it's not your job to assess their suicide risk. Ask for professional help for them and, if you need it, for you too.

To summarise, we have now outlined two parts of the answer to the question 'why self-harm?' We have talked about the distinction (uncertain as it sometimes is) between attempted suicide and self-harm without immediate suicidal intent, and we have discussed how self-harm can be both a symptom of and a response to distress. In the next chapter I want to complete the picture by touching on the idea that self-harm can have some helpful functions as a coping mechanism.

chapter 5

Are there ever positive reasons to self-harm?

I think you can guess what my answer to this question is going to be. If I thought the answer was 'No' then I wouldn't be writing a whole chapter about it. First, let's start with a clear rebuttal of one idea. When I talk about 'positive reasons', I am definitely *not* suggesting that people self-harm because they find it enjoyable (we'll come to this idea later), or want to manipulate other people or simply because they like to shock others. So what do I mean?

Many years of clinical practice, whether in outpatient clinics, hospital wards or emergency departments, has taught me that to understand any emotional problem it is not enough just to grasp fully what is happening in the present. You have to go back in time to explore the moment when it started.

With self-harm, you have to look back at when it started in exactly the same way. What I have found in talking to people who self-harm is that their first episodes were always in response to distress. But over time, if the self-harm is repeated, something changes: it comes to serve a purpose for the individual that goes beyond its original function as a coping mechanism. It is doing something else that is less closely related to relieving distress. After all, in pretty much all aspects of life we only keep doing something (assuming we have a choice) because there's something in it for us. As humans, we generally stop doing anything if it is not working for us. If the self-harm is not directly relieving the distress it must be doing something else, or it would fade away as a regular action.

Recently a student in my department at the University of Leeds undertook a project that illustrates this point, looking at social media postings tagged as 'self-harm'. One of the findings that is particularly interesting is how commonly the language of addiction cropped up. Posts talked about the struggle not to go back to the habit of self-harm, or celebrated spells of being 'clear'. It was evident that repeated self-harm has a positive draw, and that some people identify very strongly with it.

This isn't to suggest that people do this 'for kicks' or 'for fun'. That sort of dismissive thinking would indicate prejudice and lack of understanding. To be truly compassionate, and to help the person find their way out of this miserable condition, it is important to know what you are working with, and the contradictory motivations that shape human behaviour need to be understood in order to move forward.

So, without judging, it's important to note that for some who do it repeatedly, self-harm seems to offer a positive experience. This falls into two main areas of life, long after self-harm started as a response to stress:

◆ The actual experience of the self-harm itself can become (surprisingly) positive.

◆ Self-harm can become something that defines who you are as a person – which is important for people who overwhelmingly see themselves in a negative light.

These positive reasons go hand in hand with the negative reasons that always underlie self-harm, so to talk about them isn't a way of saying that self-harm is a great thing to do. Of course it would be better if nobody wanted to self-harm, but thinking about what may be positive reasons can help us to understand why people may find it difficult to stop. Before going on to unpack these ideas and explain them, it's important to emphasise that these 'positive' aspects of self-harm are really only significant for people who repeatedly self-harm. One-off acts are almost always part of a response to distress. The main exception to this is a relatively unusual (but important to recognise) situation where someone, only once in their life, harms themselves as an experimental act 'just to see what it's like'. If you know that this is what your loved one has done, or realise that it is what you have done yourself, it can be a great relief to put it behind you and to get on with your life. In such a case, it is not a question of suicidal intent or part of a pattern of distress. One-off events just happen and you move on. This chapter concerns people who repeatedly harm themselves.

Self-harm as a positive experience

A sense of control

What could anyone say about self-harm that would make you think it has a positive effect for the person doing it? Probably the commonest remark people make about self-harm is that it gives them a sense of control over some aspect of their lives. This is a really important observation, especially when you consider that it comes from people who frequently regard themselves as powerless and feel hopeless about shaping their lives.

I've noticed how reluctant people are to stop self-harm even when they have come asking for help. It's as if they think you're trying to take something away from them that's theirs. They'll make it clear you can't control what they do – it's their decision. It can feel frustrating but I also get that they need that to have that sense of control nobody can take away.

Psychiatric nurse therapist

A sense of strength or power

Reflect for a moment – swallowing poisonous doses of drugs is a risky business. Not everybody can take the risk. Cutting or burning yourself hurts. Not everybody can take the pain. Sometimes those who can do either of these things get a sense of something like achievement when they reflect on it – not like gloating or pride but an awareness that any means of survival in adversity takes some resilience.

When I think about what I've done to myself by self-harming I know that I've done something difficult and it tells me I'm stronger than other people. It reminds me that I don't have to rely on other people for support – which is good because they let you down.

Colin, 46

A sense of pleasure

We've touched on the idea that self-harm can be a way of controlling or switching off unpleasant emotions. Here I am talking about something rather different, which is the idea that self-harm can produce positively pleasurable emotions and not just help remove un-pleasurable ones. In its more extreme form, some people get a real sense of excitement or arousal from thinking about or planning an act of self-harm and then doing it. That's uncommon though, and for most people who recognise this pleasurable side it's more that they get a sense of something pleasant emotionally or physically.

I always know when I am going to do something – I think about it all day at work, what I'll do, and I picture it in my mind's eye. It sort of builds up like a tension, but a nice tension. It can feel quite exciting in a way. When I've done it, if it doesn't hurt too much or make too much mess, I can just lie back and relax ... It's like a comfortable feeling ... warm I suppose, calm like lying in a warm bath.

Joanna, 23

Very occasionally this sense of build-up, excitement and then release can be experienced as akin to sexual arousal. This isn't common, but it does happen for some people and can be built into their sexual behaviour.

Self-harm as protective

Most people who harm themselves feel vulnerable in their lives – unsure about other people, afraid of being hurt emotionally or physically, not sure if anybody really cares for them. How can self-harm help that feeling?

As a psychiatrist, I struggled sometimes to understand how self-harm could make somebody feel safer. Sophie explained it to me like this when I saw her in my clinic:

I like the feeling I get from caring for myself afterwards. If I've cut myself, I'll clean and dry the wound and take care over it. If I've taken tablets, even if I still feel miserable, I will go to bed and curl up in the warmth under my duvet. It isn't everything but it's me looking after myself, just in a small way and just for a while.

Sophie, 22

We saw earlier that self-harm and aggression sometimes go together, and in those circumstances I have met people (usually men) who use self-harm in a quite deliberate way to stop themselves from harming other people.

At times I feel so angry I just have to do something. I think if I let it go then I could kill somebody – I wouldn't know when to stop. I know what I'm capable of – my last trouble was when I hit this bloke who'd accidently knocked into

me in the post office. He needed hospital treatment and that
was my second lot of time. If I can't do it any other way
I'll break things at home or put a window in or punch the
wall. Once I put my arm through a window and had to have
fifteen stitches. I meant to do it and it got rid of the anger.

Alf, 53, has spent several years in prison

Self-harm as defining who you are

What I am talking about here is the difficult idea of a
sense of identity. What does it mean to say that somebody doesn't know who they are, or that they have a
weak sense of identity that can be bolstered by doing
something like harming themselves?

Obviously, I don't mean literally that they don't
know who they are – what their name is, where they
live, what job they have, and so on. I mean something
more subtle about what defines us as individuals. What
might that be like?

◆ A sense of having a meaningful existence – being
something to other people so that you 'exist' for them
even when you're not around. That feeling can't be
strong if you don't believe anybody cares about you or
respects you.

◆ A sense of fitting in, being like other people rather
than a misfit oddity 'from another planet'. That sense
of fitting in must be hard to maintain if you've never
had a close friend, belonged to a social group or had a
stable loving family life.

◆ A sense of being able to communicate with other people, 'speaking their language' emotionally as well as literally. That sense is difficult to develop if you have never had an intimate relationship (sexual or not) or if nobody has ever helped you express how you feel.

◆ A sense of your own body as something that defines you. Years of sexual or physical abuse can teach you that your body isn't yours to manage at all, that it is at the mercy of the whims or desires of others, and that you have no say.

Self-harm and a sense of meaningfulness

This idea of feeling that you *are* somebody, that you matter in the world, is one that people who self-harm seem to find particularly difficult to express.

It's like when I harm myself then it says, everything I've been through is real and understandable. When I tell other people, it's like 'this is who I am, I'm struggling but I'm a survivor'. If they don't like it I can understand that – it's scary and unfamiliar to them. But it's me and I'm real and I'm here so at least that's something that makes me feel my feet are on the ground.

Jack, 38

Self-harm and belonging

While some people who harm themselves feel very alone with it, lots of people – and especially younger people – know that there are others doing the same thing. Social media has helped in that way (there is more on social media later in the book). There are groups that are defined by self-harming, typically using online forums, and there are groups for whom self-harm is just accepted if not encouraged.

It just felt good to be accepted, you know? Not to have to hide it. To be able to … hey I cut myself … and nobody freaks.

Josh, 19

Self-harm as a personal language

Sometimes self-harm means something that can't be put into words. At times that meaning is not too difficult to grasp; scars remind people of a specific event or of their journey in life to get where they are today. So scars can act as a prompt to remembrance, helping to conjure up good memories or good feelings about personal resilience.

I touch this and I know when I did it, and I'm not in that place now. But all that stuff made me who I am today and I'm a strong person so it speaks to me, it's like an entry in my diary. I'm not ashamed of it, it's part of who I am.

Sophie, 32 (touching the scar on her forearm)

These ideas about self-harm – defining something about who you are, being meaningful in a personal way that you can't put into words – aren't easy to get across. People who self-harm are often trying to convey something like this but they may struggle to put it into words, as of course it can be a struggle for any of us to find the right words for how we feel.

Self-harm and the body

Most of us have a sense of personal space. It's outside our skin but it's still 'part' of us. People who stand inside it or touch us uninvited can feel invasive. It can be good to assert these boundaries every so often (sadly, especially for women): 'Please don't stand so close, you're making me feel uncomfortable.' Suppose you didn't have such a good sense of where your boundaries were? How could you establish them and assert yourself as a physical person? One way might be to mark your skin so that both the act of doing it and the physical evidence afterwards serve as a sign. For example, self-cutting has been described as 'writing on the skin' and some people do indeed write words. A few people make patterns with repeated cuts. This can be a way of saying: 'This is my body, I can choose how I use my skin, these scars are personal to me.'

*

Although the above illustrates some aspects of what can be experienced as the positive functions of self-harm, it is not, essentially, a positive experience to harm yourself. Fundamentally self-harm is a sign of, and response to, distress. It is something we should see as worthy of attention and a sign that understanding and support is needed.

The next part of the book discusses some approaches to managing or getting help. The ideas we've covered so far will crop up again as we look at some of these strategies.

part three

What help is there for self-harm?

chapter 6

What can you do to help yourself?

This chapter is mainly for those readers who harm themselves. The suggestions aren't just about ways of stopping your self-harming. They are also about how you can start on the road to feeling better about yourself. If you are a friend or family member of somebody who self-harms you may also find some of this useful so that you can provide support to the person you know.

Remember: nothing in self-harm applies to everybody so don't be downhearted if you don't find what you want here, or if you feel that you've tried this already and it did not help. Sometimes it's worth going back to things you've tried before – it is important to have another go. The fact that you are reading this means that you want to be well, and to be well it is vital that you try things rather than giving up. Think of it as an experiment. And remember that it's not a catastrophe if it doesn't work. Tell yourself : 'I am not a personal failure just because this one thing doesn't work for me. It was worth a try.'

If you really feel that you have tried as hard as you can and gone as far as you can with trying to help yourself, and you are still in trouble, you must get help. There are later chapters on how to seek outside help.

You can think about self-help in three areas if you like:

◆ Looking after yourself – the basics of self-care

◆ What to do in a crisis

◆ Moving towards longer-term change.

Looking after yourself – five tips for self-care

Self-harm and the problems that go with it seem so big that it's difficult to know where to start. Suggesting some basic attention to your lifestyle can seem trivial or dismissive.

When I saw my GP he said I should try and keep more regular hours and eat a healthier diet. I mean … I've been harming myself since I was 14 and I've been in hospital twice after overdoses. How is going to bed early like a good girl going to help?

Myrna, 22

Well, of course, improving your lifestyle isn't going to be the whole answer. But a few simple steps can have two benefits. First, there is good evidence that the lifestyle changes described below can have a positive effect on mood.

Second, and perhaps more importantly, by making these small changes you are giving the message to yourself that you are worth the effort. When you acknowledge that these small steps are worthwhile you are starting to overcome the black and white way of thinking that says, 'If I can't change the big problems in my life then it's not worth doing anything at all.' Even if your progress is slow, you are still making progress as long as you change something, however small.

1. *Think about what you eat*

   We can all recognise the affect that food has on our moods – how grumpy we can get when we're hungry, or how some food fills us up while other food makes us feel bloated or dissatisfied. This is not to promote a patented self-harm prevention diet – just to note that most people feel better if they eat a balanced mixture of foods, cut down on processed food and try to eat regular meals.

   The point of these steps towards change isn't about diet alone, it's also about starting to think about making small changes in your life, changes over which you have some control. These may be small steps but if they are achievable then they are better than overambitious attempts at major change all in one leap. So don't just think about *what* you eat but about *how* you eat. Try to avoid snacking in the kitchen, always sit down at a table to eat, even if it's just a tea-time snack, and preferably don't eat in front of the TV.

   If you eat for comfort and have put on too much weight as a result of being unhappy, don't try crash diets or fad diets and don't beat yourself up about it.

There is lots of information available about what a balanced diet is if you look up 'healthy eating' on websites such as NHS Choices, and recipes on the BBC Good Food website. There are some simple steps you can take to start out:

◆ Have some ready-prepared healthy snacks available – peel whatever fruit or vegetables you like and keep a supply in the fridge.

◆ Keep cold water or unsweetened fruit juice in a bottle in the fridge.

◆ If you don't already, try to find the time to make yourself a proper meal (rather than a snack) every so often.

2. *Control your use of alcohol and recreational drugs*

A recent research study showed that one of the three things that made a difference to self-harm rates was giving up alcohol. The role of alcohol and drugs in self-harm is widely recognised.

Our records show that nearly half of all the people who come here for treatment after self-harm have been drinking or smoking weed (cannabis) in the hours before they harmed. They aren't really badly intoxicated but it must play a role.

Senior nurse in the emergency department

This may be because alcohol and drugs are both mood-altering and can often contribute to sudden dips. If you drink alcohol or use drugs you should consider stopping or cutting down. It's a good idea not to drink alcohol on your own, particularly when you are feeling miserable.

3. *Try to keep physically active*

What you do depends on where you are starting from. If you are already used to exercising, or feel ready for more activity, then you might choose to go for a run in your local park, try some yoga at home or even go to the gym. If you feel unfit, or unable to go straight to these options, then you can still benefit from doing something relatively light, like going for a short walk. There is good evidence that exercise can help lift mood. It can also act to build in a break from more isolated activities and help you interrupt a stream of negative thoughts.

While one-off activities can lift mood, to really feel the benefit of exercise long term, it's important to make it a regular part of your life. This is hard to do simply by giving yourself a pep talk. You need a plan. Start in small ways. First, think about how you could build more activity into your daily routine – get off the bus a stop early and walk the last bit home, take the stairs rather than the lift. Second, schedule some extra activity in your life: you could sign up for a class (like salsa or Pilates – whatever tempts you), or pick one day a week for a jog. It can be helpful to keep a diary – when are there times in your day when you are both (a) physically inactive, and (b) not enjoying yourself that much? Even a ten-minute walk in those times is better than sitting around. Small changes are possible.

4. *Be careful about listening to music*

Music has mood-altering effects. Like alcohol, how music affects you can depend on what mood you start off in. We each have our preferences so I won't name names, but some music can make us feel calm, while other kinds can make us feel more miserable. You will know what has an effect on you.

I really always liked [names band] and I saw them live twice. But now if I listen there's something about it that brings me down ... maybe it's the lyrics, maybe it reminds me of happier times. Whatever, I have learned that I just had better not listen to them when I am on my own and feeling off it anyway.

Dean, 32

So if you listen to music a lot, get to know what sort of music lifts your mood or calms you, and what makes you feel more sad or lonely. Don't listen to the second sort of music when you are on your own or already feeling low.

5. *Fix yourself small treats*

This isn't a 'Don't worry, be happy' message. Treats don't always help, but just doing something for yourself is a message about your value. Decide in what small ways you will spoil yourself – favourite places to visit or films to watch, favourite things to eat or drink, places to go for a walk or just sit. Just try them every so often – it doesn't have to be when you need cheering up, it can be when you feel you are most likely to enjoy your treat.

The point is to do something for yourself of no great significance – just something for you!

When I asked her if she ever felt happy, Maxine told me:

It's a funny thing … at big events like weddings or family get-togethers when everyone is happy I just feel nervous. Out of place. But small things, I can sometimes enjoy them. If I have a bit of money and I'm in town I will buy myself an expensive hot chocolate and just sit on my own with it. It just feels good for that while with nobody to please but myself.

Maxine, 43

Sometimes, people who aren't working and are receiving benefits, especially for mental health problems, can feel guilty about treating themselves. If this applies to you then think of treats as part of a rehab programme in order to challenge that guilt. You do deserve it.

What to do in a crisis – three tips

'Crisis' means a situation that calls for some quick response from you because it is affecting your emotional state. For example, you might have hit unexpected financial problems with debts you can't meet, or a relationship has broken up or threatens to, or you have been involved in an unpleasant scene at work about which you feel bad. Two of the following suggestions aren't specific at all to self-harm and the third one is. The main message here is: make yourself a crisis plan. It can be difficult to think clearly once a crisis has struck and it's much better to have the basic steps of what to do worked out in advance. If you can guess what the next crisis might be (because the same issue keeps cropping up) then your plan might be quite specific, but you can still make some general plans about what to do even if what happens is completely unexpected. Perhaps in discussion with somebody you trust write down your plan; keep it where it's easy to find (and ideally somewhere it's difficult to ignore). What should be in your plan?

1. *Take steps to slow down the action*

What is meant by 'slowing down the action'? It's a way of saying 'don't act impulsively'. Stop and think it through. When I was working in acute hospital medicine a colleague used to say, 'What we need to do here is feed in some time', meaning – 'Hardly anything is an emergency. You don't always have to act at once. Avoid panicky actions by waiting until it's clear about what the right thing to do is.'

How do you go about feeding in some time? The answer is to take it in steps.

The first step is to ask: what exactly is the problem? If it's something somebody has said, why does it bother you so much? Perhaps it brings back bad memories or you feel angry or let down. Perhaps you are worried about the longer-term consequences of what's happened. Try to put what has happened into some perspective. How does it compare to other problems you've had? Can you think of other ways you could understand the situation? Write down the problem as it is for you, not just what happened.

Anita is upset by the way her daughter Nicola speaks to her. In their latest argument her daughter called her a useless mother and stormed off. After thinking about it, Anita wrote down the problem for her:

1. Being called a useless mother reminds me of the sadness I had from growing up with my own mum, who drank too much and neglected us.

2. When Nicola says things like that to me I worry that I am not bringing her up well and whether she's right: I am a useless mother.

3. Nicola is getting to be a teenager and I don't know how to help her control her temper and lead a happy life as she gets older.

The advantage of this way of thinking is that it suggests to Anita what she can do next. But ... it takes practice to do this.

Take time to think through your problem – not going over what happens (rehearsing your problems in your head) but trying to understand it. Imagine how it would seem to somebody else. For example, Anita tried to think about what Nicola felt like and concluded that she might ask herself 'Why is Mum always so cross with me?' That helped Anita to think 'Yes, why am I so cross with her? Is it just about her or is it about me as well? This 'reversing roles' can be a useful way of seeing a problem from a different angle.

Once you have had a go at describing your problems and picked one you want to work on, the second step is to ask yourself: are there some different solutions to try? You might come up with some solutions simply by sitting down and jotting down every possible thing you can think of – even if to start it seems silly. Then pick one or two. Or you could talk through options with a friend or (if you have one) a counsellor.

Anita thought of three solutions she could try.

1. Dealing with sad memories rather than tackling Nicola. This will help her see that some of her emotional troubles come not from Nicola's behaviour but from her own earlier life.

2. Writing a reminder list of the ways she had chosen to be a mother unlike her own mother – for example, cooking family meals, not drinking, not smacking her children.

3. Arranging to have a chat with Nicola about something enjoyable they could do together, and maybe have a mum-and-daughter chat at the same time.

The third step is to pick one solution to try first

– one of Anita's problems was always trying to fix everything at once. This is where you need to 'feed in some time': don't rush at the first solution that occurs to you but spend a while thinking about it – perhaps park it and come back to it later. You may decide on a particular solution because it's easy, or because you know somebody will help you with it, or because it tackles something that's important to you. Anita chose number (3) because it felt like something she could do without starting another row, and she and Nicola went to the cinema together.

2. *Try to make sure you have company and support*

    People who self-harm frequently say that there is nobody they know who will be there for them when they are low and alone, but if pressed what they often really mean is that there's no one they can bring themselves to ask. They just assume that no one will want to help or they feel ashamed about imposing on people. In some cases they will have confided in someone about their self-harm and been put off by the response. With a bit of reflection they can see that the response was, in fact, understandable, because the person they spoke to was shocked about somebody they knew self-harming. All the same they never went back to see if their confidant, after getting over the initial surprise or dismay, might indeed be able to help.

    Find somebody, or more than one person if you possibly can, who you can call on at short notice for support. I know it isn't that easy to approach another person about your problems, and if you don't feel able to tell them about your self-harm, you can tell part of the story without telling untruths – for example, saying that you suffer with spells of low mood and at those times need company. Later in this chapter I'll talk more about how to plan a conversation when you are thinking of confiding in another person about your self-harm.

What about using social media as a source of support? If you search for posts tagged as self-harm on any of several popular sites it is easy to find dozens of them. You may find that this way of confiding suits you – it allows you to share while keeping it all at a distance.

Like everything else, you might want to give it a try, but there are some basic rules:

◆ Avoid posting personal details or photographs that make you identifiable.

◆ Remember that you never really know who you are talking to. Most estimates suggest that at least 10 per cent of posters on the common social media sites are using fake names or multiple accounts.

◆ Don't get drawn in by sites that encourage self-harm or try to set up a view of the world that promotes 'us-against-them' attitudes. They aren't very common but if you do find one be aware that these people don't know you or care about you. They are just on their own self-absorbed trip and may take pleasure from encouraging others to harm.

◆ Be very careful about looking at images of self-harm. It's not difficult to find lurid pictures but these have nothing to tell you about your own problems.

◆ Be prepared to be surprised or disappointed at the content. Some of it is obviously about self-harm but you'll find posts about fashion, eating disorders, or people's pets.

◆ Find some real-life company if you have been upset by something you have seen on social media. You don't have to explain what's happened (although it might help if you tried): all you need is time with somebody to help you stop brooding about what you've encountered.

If you do look at social media you'll find both encouraging stories about improvement and dispiriting stories about the lack of it. Don't try to identify too closely with any of it. Remember the advice elsewhere in this book: in the world of self-harm there is no single thing that applies to everybody, because we are all different.

3. *Consider substituting self-harm with another action*

Sometimes you will read suggestions about actions to interrupt or replace self-harm. These are things you can do straight away, without relying on other people, and that don't need a lot of forward planning. They might be agreeable things like taking a warm bath. They might be disagreeable things that at least are not damaging, like taking a freezing cold shower or squeezing ice cubes. Or they might mimic something harmful you are trying to avoid, such as drawing red lines on your skin instead of cutting.

Not everybody likes the idea of substitutes. These suggestions can sound trivialising – it can seem rather patronising or dismissive to say 'Why don't you do this instead?' as if a simple substitution could sort things out. On the other hand, it's a useful attitude to have that if you want to try something, you should go for it. So, if you don't think it sounds right for you, that's fine. If you do and it helps you even a little, then good. If it doesn't help, you will at least have learned something and there's nothing lost from having tried.

Mike and Toni were discussing this issue in a self-help group. Mike said 'I tried smacking an elastic band against my wrist until it hurt but to be honest I just thought it was a bit silly. I know what it was supposed to be doing, but it's not the real deal, is it?' Toni disagreed. 'I know what you mean, and I felt like that, but a friend suggested drawing red lines on my arm. I was surprised but it helped a bit. It doesn't sort it all out but it was just another small helpful thing to do.'

Moving towards longer-term change

This chapter is about ways in which you can help yourself, and doing so is an important part of making change. However, it's not all down to you. Change is hard and outside help is of value to all of us. In this section, we'll look at what you might do to prepare yourself for getting that help, or going back for another try if you have been for help before and yet still have problems. Here are three tips for getting ready for longer-term change.

1. *Take stock – are you ready?*

Perhaps the place to start is to ask yourself a difficult and challenging question. How much do you really want to change and to stop self-harming? Maybe you have been doing it for some time. Maybe it feels like something that is 'yours' and you don't want to risk it being taken away with nothing put in its place.

I know in a way that I ought to try and stop it. I mean, it's not normal, is it? It stops me making relationships and that. But when I get down to it I think, even when I saw a therapist, like, 'This is me, I'm not going to let you stop me.' It's like the first thing I've got to do is want to want-to-stop, if you know what I mean.

Suzanne, 33

Here's one way that might help to think about motivation. Think of two people: 'My ideal me, the me I'd like to be' and 'The actual me, who I am.' Don't run yourself down by comparison with some unattainable fantasy person, just think about the changed person you might imagine it possible to be. Now think: 'What reasons are there to be like the ideal me?' Often, people come up with a long list of answers to that question, but if there were really that many reasons to be different and so few reasons to stay as they are, they'd have changed by now. Sometimes the barriers to change are outside in the world, but sometimes they are in you. You might want to stay as you are because it's familiar (all change can be threatening), or because it's something you can control, whereas changing to be different feels like taking on something unknown: you might lose good things along with the bad things you would like to change. So, you need to think again about reasons for trying to change and reasons for not changing.

This exercise is challenging, and it won't change your life, but it may help you to think about what you have to face in order to take on the changes you're aiming for.

2. *Think about the people in your life*

Think about the people who form your network of family, friends and acquaintances. Is there somebody you can confide in? Don't give up too soon on this, even if you've tried before or think there is no one. Make a list, including people you have talked to before about other (perhaps more minor) problems or people you know are sympathetic or understanding, or who you are confident won't talk to others without your permission. Sometimes you may want to talk to somebody who you feel has a duty to help you. Here are some ideas about planning the conversation if you do decide to confide in somebody.

◆ Think about who you will tell and why. Do you want to pick somebody practical, and perhaps a bit unemotional, who won't freak out about what you tell them? Or somebody you have seen be sympathetic in another situation? Or somebody in your family, because you don't think it's fair for them not to know? Who you choose is up to you, but it may help to be clear about why.

◆ Plan a time and place for your conversation. Don't just start on the spur of the moment. You can say something like 'I'd like to talk to you about something personal, can we sit and talk/meet on Tuesday morning?'

◆ Decide how much you want to say and set yourself a clear limit to what you want to confide – especially at a first meeting. Don't just blurt out everything that comes to mind once you start. Better to say too little at first, but in a clear way, than to start with a rush and not know how to manage the conversation. You can stop by saying 'That's all I want to say for now, if you don't mind' or something similar.

◆ Don't imagine, in advance, your ideal response. You may get pretty much the response you expected, or you may be surprised and get a disappointing or negative response. This is more likely if you talk to somebody because you think they *should* help, rather than because they have behaved in the past as if they will help. The one time I think you can be fairly sure about what will happen is this – if you decide to confront somebody who has treated you badly or abused you in some way you can be pretty certain that you won't get an acknowledgement or apology, at least at a first talk. So, be ready for anything – the point at this stage is to start the conversation.

◆ Plan what you are going to say about why you have chosen to confide. Do you have something specific you want to ask for, like company to go to a clinic? Or do you, for now, just want to reduce the sense of coping with something on your own? If the person you are speaking to doesn't feel able to do exactly what you want, don't take it as an outright rejection. Try to talk about what they do feel able to offer.

◆ Unless it goes really badly, remember to say 'Thank you for listening.' It's hard for you, but it's likely to be hard for the person you're talking to as well.

◆ And remember, if things don't go well or don't go to plan don't give up after one attempt. Think how you might have handled it differently and consider going back for another try – or talking to someone else.

Suppose, after thinking carefully about it, you decide that there is nobody at all in whom you want to confide. This raises a different question: for example, perhaps you have the wrong living arrangements – with family, sharing with friends, or in a relationship. Should you move? Don't jump at it – discuss it with somebody you trust, maybe a friend outside the home, or a sibling you don't see that often, or a professional like your GP. The point is to try out the idea with someone who can give a different perspective on it. There is no need to rush, but consider that if the people in your life are part of the problem perhaps you need some distance from them. You could try it as an experiment and move back if it doesn't work out: somebody who really cares about you should be able to understand that.

I was stuck and didn't think I could manage living on my own, but when I thought about it I realised I was surrounded by my problems in the house. Every room had bad memories for me, every day I was being undermined and criticised. It felt like the only safe place was my bedroom but that started to feel like a prison. It's not perfect now but I'm glad I took that step.

Kim, 28

3. Ask yourself exactly how you'd describe your problems

See if you can try to change how you think about your problems. I mean that – not change just *what* you think about but *how* you think. Can you try to think about your past experiences without just brooding on them? One way to do that is to try to change when and how you approach thinking about your life. I often suggest to people that they write a letter if they don't find talking easy – to themselves or to somebody in their life. You don't have to send the letter for it to work.

After we spoke I wrote a letter to my uncle. I told him what an effect he'd had on my life and how angry I was that he'd died before I could confront him about it. I told him that he needed to understand that and that I didn't need to tell anybody else now because I had talked about it with another person [in therapy] and I was ready to start living my life more happily. Then I set fire to the letter and watched the smoke and heat rise. It was a strange feeling, like I was sending it to him Special Delivery and at the same time like I was finishing something just for me, or at least beginning to finish it. It definitely helped how I think about him now – he's less able to have an influence on my life.

Nancy, 42

You could also try to take a problem-solving approach to emotional challenges, a bit like Anita in the example earlier in this chapter. A problem-solving approach is when you step back and try to think how to deal with your difficulty logically, rather than responding emotionally. You can think of it as having the following steps:

1. Write a problem list – if you pick it apart, what seems like one problem may turn out to be several. This may seem like making work for yourself but in fact it will make it easier to think about solutions. Notice how Anita thought she had only one problem (arguing with her daughter) but was able to split it into three parts, each with a different solution.

2. Pick the problem you want to start with. It needn't be the most important. You might pick the easiest (quick wins will make you feel better) or the one you need to tackle soonest.

3. For your chosen problem, write a solution list. Try to think of at least three different solutions you might try. Make them specific – not 'I'll try not to shout at my sister when I am angry with her' but 'When I feel myself getting angry I will leave the room for a moment to calm down.' By the way, notice that there are two problems here – getting angry and shouting when you are angry. Taking time out is one solution to one of the problems.

4. Try out your solution– more than once if you can.

5. Afterwards, think about how it went. If it went

well, what have your learned? If it went badly, don't abandon hope. Think about how you could try the same solution but slightly differently or think about what other solution on your list you could try. The important point is to keep experimenting.

Finally, I need to say something about an important topic. Even if you would like to change you may find that it's a slow process. You have to accept where you are starting from and not be too hard on yourself if you find it difficult to make a move from there. Sometimes that includes accepting that, at least for a while, you may feel the need to continue harming yourself. Sometimes it means accepting that you will use methods to keep what harm you do under control, even if you can't stop yet. This is called *harm minimisation* or *harm reduction*. Some of the approaches suggested for harm minimisation are:

◆ Do not share blades, pins or needles with other people. There is a risk you could get an infectious disease.

◆ Don't self-harm on areas where you have lots of scars. Scar tissue may not be as strong as your skin.

◆ Learn about your body so that you can avoid doing damage to major nerves or blood vessels.

◆ Learn first aid and keep first-aid supplies nearby. Include antiseptic wipes and bandages.

◆ Have an emergency plan, such as keeping a phone nearby so that you can ring an ambulance if you need to.

◆ Set yourself limits before you self-harm and stick to them. For example, decide how many cuts you will make and how big they will be. This is a good way of learning the skills you need to stop.

◆ Think of options that don't break your skin.

I wouldn't suggest that you try this without getting some advice, especially if you are worried that you might already have done some irreversible damage. You could ask your GP or another professional you trust, or try one of the helping organisations listed at the back, like RETHINK.

In the next chapter I will talk about getting help from others. Don't forget – there is no one thing that works for everybody, and you may find that you try some of these ideas and are disappointed. In fact, you are almost certain to try something that doesn't work. Remember the experimental approach and keep going. Take a break and go back to try something again: if you or your circumstances have changed it may work this time even when it didn't before. And remember, it's not just down to you to sort it out. You are likely to need help from others and you should feel able to ask for it. That's what the next two chapters are about.

chapter 7

Friends, family and other sources of help

When people write about where to go for help for health problems, they sometimes divide it into informal help and formal help. Informal help comes from your social world. You get it from people who are not paid for their time in helping. Formal help comes from statutory bodies like the NHS and social services who are paid to provide this sort of service to people. This chapter is about informal help – the sort of help provided by those who know you as a family member or friend, or who work for a voluntary organisation.

Let's begin with tips for friends and family. What do you do when you learn that somebody you are close to is self-harming? Remember, if you are in this position, that your job isn't to be a therapist. It is not for you to assess the risk to somebody you care about or to 'go it alone' in doing something about the situation. Instead, your role is to be there to offer support and to try to help them get better while they get any formal help they need. If you are somebody who self-harms, please read this too – and try to let yourself accept genuine offers of help when they are offered.

Seven tips for helping somebody who self-harms

1. *Acknowledge how you feel yourself*

    When you learn that somebody you care about is self-harming it is natural to be upset and shocked. You might feel hurt that they didn't turn to you before, or angry about how they are behaving. You might feel guilty – 'Is it something I've done?'

    It's no good trying to pretend that you don't have those feelings; the person you are speaking to will spot them anyway. And it won't help if you express those strong feelings forcefully: all that will do is close down the discussion. Both you and the person you care for will end up feeling hurt and alone. So though it is best to speak honestly about how it makes you feel, it is really important to try to stay calm. Try pausing before you say something emotional. Say just a little at a time – don't try to get it all out at once. Pause to check how the person you are talking with is responding and let them speak when they want to, even if you feel you haven't yet finished what you want to say.

    When I first told me mum she got really upset and tearful and then after a few minutes she got angry and said 'How could you?' While I was trying to find the words to explain she calmed down and said, 'I'm sorry, I am just so upset to think about you doing this without being able to talk to me first, but I can understand how difficult it must have been to admit it.' That was just such a wonderful thing to say. I could see she was still upset, but she was on my side.

    Bill, 16

2. *Listen to the full story*

Try to get a clear picture of how the person who is self-harming feels about it, what they have done and what they want now. Ask questions gently to explore how much they want to tell you, but don't interrogate them.

The first time I told somebody it was my friend and it was awful. She just kept asking 'Why?' And I'd say I don't know and she said 'You must know' and then she wanted to know what I'd done and if I had any scars and she wanted to look at my arms. It was like it wasn't about me and what mattered to me at all. Later, when I told my sister, she was much better, just waited for me to say as much as I wanted and encouraged me to talk without pressing me.

Shahana, 24

Perhaps the most difficult part of a conversation about mental health comes in talking with somebody who has ideas about suicide. As noted before, it's not your job to make an assessment of suicide risk – but at the same time you don't want to just change the subject or act as if this is something you just can't talk about. We know that many people in distress have thoughts of suicide and it's no bad thing to acknowledge that. Here are a few tips about what you might talk about, to help you and the person you are with face this difficult topic:

◆ The nature of thoughts about suicide can vary from passing thoughts, to plans, to definite actions. Are any of these thoughts just fleeting, quickly pushed away, or are they more like painful preoccupations?

Have the thoughts led to plans about what to do? Has any action been taken about these plans, for example saving tablets or checking out how to use certain methods?

◆ Suppose the person you are talking with hasn't got as far as making plans but is definitely having suicidal thoughts. Can they say what they think about acting on those ideas? Is it something that they think they might do some time or is it an immediate issue? Can they say what would stop them? (Often it's the thoughts about how others would feel that makes someone stop.)

◆ If you are worried by this discussion and asking yourself how safe the person is, then say something about it. There's no harm in acknowledging how you feel, and it might lead to a helpful move into planning what to do next. You can explain how much you don't want somebody to kill themselves without just pressing them for reassurance for yourself.

◆ Talk about what you can both do about any suicidal thoughts. What's the best way to feel safe when they do come? Do you know who to call in a crisis – either friend or family, or one of the organisations listed at the end of this book?

It's best, if at all possible, not to try to do things in this situation without involving the person who has self-harmed. They may feel let down rather than supported and might not trust you again with their confiding. However, it may be that you feel you just *have* to do something, for the safety of somebody you care about.

For ideas about what to do you should read the next chapter on getting help from the health service. Try not to keep it a secret – nobody can reasonably blame you for doing what you think is for the best and even if it provokes an angry response initially, it is likely to be appreciated later.

Sometimes, you know, we have to respond to risk in this situation by doing something our patients don't want. My experience is that, in the end, most people don't harbour resentment if they know you have acted in what you genuinely thought were their best interests. What does cause resentment is a sense that you've acted to cover your own back (against complaints in case anything happens).

Dr E, a psychiatrist, discussing suicide risk

3. *Be clear about what you can do to help*

It's most likely that you have found out about this because the person who self-harms has told you themselves, but are you aware of their reasons for speaking to you specifically? Don't make assumptions – ask.

First off I was just shocked when he told me, he just didn't seem that sort of bloke. When he started telling me about it I realised he'd been hiding a lot about how he felt, like putting on a jokey who-cares-about-anything act. While we were talking I thought – I wonder why he's telling me? So I asked him. He said he'd noticed how I talked about my sister's troubles (she has just left a violent partner) and he thought I'd be sympathetic. There was a pause and I thought – OK, I am sympathetic but what can I do? So I

asked him and we got talking about if I'd go with him to see
somebody about getting help.

Danny, talking about his friend Joe

At the same time be clear about what you feel you can offer. It may be less than is asked for, or simply different. This may sound like rejection to somebody who finds it difficult to ask for help, so try to have a discussion about what's realistic for both of you – a shared plan is likely to last whereas a plan based on conditions set by one party only is likely to fall apart. Don't feel guilty about acknowledging your own needs in this situation – you can only do what is practical given your own circumstances.

4. *Have a think (and talk) about who needs to know*

Confidentiality is really important in health issues, especially those issues that might be shocking or embarrassing. Every adult has a perfect right to decide to keep their health details to themselves and not share them with others. Put simply, they have the mental ability to make their own decisions and the right to have their decisions about their information respected. That ability is called 'mental capacity' or just 'capacity'. An adult is anyone over 16 years of age but the capacity to make decisions actually starts before then. So the person who confides in you can decide that no one else should know, even close family or the people they are living with. Of course you might think that it's not a good idea for them to keep it to themselves in this way, but it's not your decision.

You certainly shouldn't tell lots of people just because you are worried. You are likely to lose the trust of the person who has confided in you and you may not do them any good.

In the example above, I asked Danny about Joe's family. He said that he'd asked Joe and that Joe had said definitely not to talk to his family. Joe said that if Danny told them, then he wouldn't come to the clinic. Danny didn't tell Joe's family, although he was worried about keeping secrets – he and Joe had known each other since primary school. I made a note to myself that it was something I needed to talk to Joe about when he was ready.

There's an exception to this rule. If you are seriously worried that somebody is thinking of taking their own life, then you should act. This is especially important if you think that they have a mental health problem that is affecting their judgement. Then (but only then) you should tell someone else who you can enlist to help. If you think that someone you know is actively suicidal then what they need is professional help. If you are worried that something needs to be done urgently, remember that there is always 24-hour emergency cover from the NHS. You can make contact if you call your GP's number at any time; if the surgery is closed it will transfer you or tell you what number to call. You can also dial NHS 24 on 111: many local mental health services run a 24-hour crisis number you can call for advice – NHS 24 or the 24/7 general practice service should be able to give you the number. There are several crisis lines run by voluntary organisations: see the details at the back of this book.

5. *Encourage the person you are with to seek further help*

By a long way, most people who harm themselves are not mentally ill. Nevertheless, everybody should have at least two pieces of professional help. The first is an assessment by a health professional of the nature of any mental health problems and of suicide risk. The second is a discussion with a mental health professional about whether some form of therapy might be beneficial.

This creates problems. People don't like the idea of being 'assessed' as if they can't judge for themselves how they are. Although it is the job of psychiatrists (mental health doctors) to help, most people initially don't want to see a mental health professional. They worry about stigma, being labelled, or being pressurised into having treatments they don't want. For some who do have contact with the mental health services it can be, or has been in the past, a bruising experience.

After I took the overdose I was seen in the hospital by a psychiatrist before I could go home. It was like he was sat there with a checklist on a clipboard – he couldn't have been less interested in me as a person and I could tell he just switched off halfway through when he decided I wasn't going to kill myself. He just said 'Go and see your GP' when I asked what to do next.

Annabel, 38

It is worth persisting, though. You might expect that every healthcare professional is always just that, professional: every job has good and bad workers, and every worker has good and bad days. These negative experiences are down to the nature of individual practitioners, so don't give up. Try to persuade the person who has self-harmed that it is worth trying again.

A very difficult question arises about what you should do if you really think your friend or family member needs professional help but they won't accept it. Don't try to push it or railroad them – all you will do is provoke resistance and make it less likely that they will agree. Actually, if you *do* force them along to see somebody, it is unlikely to be a success. Take your time, raise the question every so often, and maybe it will be better received over time as you increase the confidence they have in your good intention to help them be happier and healthier. You can only really go over a person's head and insist that they see someone if you believe them to be so ill that their judgement is impaired. If you are not sure what to do in this situation you might find it helpful to seek advice from your GP or one of the organisations listed at the back of this book.

6. *Find out more yourself about self-harm*

Self-harm is one of those topics about which few people are well informed but on which everybody has an opinion. Don't listen to most of those opinions: they are typically based upon no experience at all, or the experience of one case, which might even be the person themselves. You've made a start by reading this book. There are other reasonably reliable sources of information – some are mentioned below – and if you still have questions you could try one of the helplines that are now available.

7. *Be prepared for change not to come easily*

Finally, in this section, I should mention one other topic. You need to be ready for how you feel if all your efforts don't lead to an obvious change – or if they actually seem to be resisted or unwanted. That can make you feel frustrated or angry or upset. How can you help somebody who won't help themselves? You might think: 'Is it something I've done, a way of getting at me?' These and many other thoughts may occur. Such thoughts and feelings are only natural and you should accept them for what they are. What is important, however, is not to reject the person who is self-harming. That can require patience and acceptance, even if you find understanding difficult.

Sometimes I just think – why do I keep trying to help? She doesn't want it … perhaps I'll just leave her to it. And then I think – I don't love her for what she does, I love her for who she is, my daughter. She just is … I just have to be there. So that's all I can do sometimes … be there.

> Jane, mother of Susan who has been self-harming for eight years

If this is your situation then an important element of what you can do is to make sure you have your own source of emotional and perhaps practical support – somebody you can turn to. They don't even have to know everything: don't feel that you must explain it all, especially if they also know the person who self-harms but don't know all the details. It is enough that they are able to support you.

What other help is available?

It's important, first of all, to talk about help in the school or college environment, or in the workplace. Much of the information in this book so far still applies if you find out about self-harm in these more formal settings, but there are some extra considerations.

First, if you work in a school, college or in any organisation that deals with young or vulnerable people, what you do will be the subject of that organisation's policies and especially their safeguarding policy, which you will need to know and act within. For example, a policy is likely to explain the rules about who you should tell if you learn something significant about one of the students, employees or volunteers. If someone confides in you about their self-harm and you are required to tell another responsible person, then it is best to make that clear from the outset. Sometimes this information is set out in leaflets or in online information about the service. Sometimes you will just have to make it clear during your conversation.

I liked Mr Clarke at college. One day when we were in class alone he noticed a scar on my arm and asked me how I'd done it so I told him I'd done it myself and about the problem I had with depression. I was really shocked when I

*discovered he'd told Mrs Lidgett and when I asked he said
he had to because of the college's safeguarding policy. I wish
he'd told me before – I'd have understood, but like this I felt
as if he hadn't been open with me like I had with him*

Emma, 23

Second, it may be that you are a member of a professional body that sets standards of behaviour. These professional standards will generally support a response from you that is helpful. You need to be clear what they are and whether they set guidance for you in this situation.

There is a lot of interest now in the planning of support in schools and colleges for students with mental health problems. This can be a good thing if, for example, it feels less scary and official than going to see a doctor. But it can feel like a bad thing if the person concerned worries about the school knowing too much about them or interfering in their private behaviour. The most important thing is to be aware of what's available and how it can be accessed, and to make sure that the person who has self-harmed is directly involved in any decision about what to do.

Finally, one of the challenges in this situation is that you may have conflicting responsibilities. As an employer or team leader your responsibility is to the organisation; as a colleague or supervisor it might also be to the person who has told you about their self-harm.

For example, doctors and nurses can have mental health problems too, and as a consultant in the NHS I had a responsibility to consider whether a colleague with mental health problems was fit to work. I could usually make this decision quite easily – the best way to judge someone's work suitability is to judge their work. But occasionally I wasn't sure. In that situation, the best arrangement is to separate the two functions – with one person caring for the individual in distress, and another making decisions about their current position in work or study. If you need to do something like this, then you need to discuss it twice with the person who self-harms, initially explaining your thinking and what you plan to do in approaching another colleague, then again to introduce that colleague and explain who has what role.

Help from voluntary organisations

At the back of this book you will find details about several organisations that offer advice and support. Some of them are set up specifically for young people; some offer help to people with a mental health problem; some are specifically for people who are feeling suicidal. Probably the best known is Samaritans, a widely used and well thought of organisation that has for many years been offering support to people, provided by trained volunteers. There are others. Don't worry if you are not sure whether it's right to contact one of them – just go for it. And remember:

- ◆ They are all confidential – you don't have to give any personal details that could identify you.
- ◆ They have been set up to help people with your sort of problems so they are staffed by people who want to help. You won't be thought of as a time-waster.

◆ They will be able to give you advice about what to do now and how to get further help

◆ Even though they are national organisations, they may have local contacts or they will advise you how to find out about local help.

I don't want to recommend one of these organisations as better than the others and I don't want to promise that any of them will definitely help you. But many people have found them helpful and you should always be willing to try new approaches and see if they are for you. If they are, good. If they are not, it's not your fault, and there are more organisations that you might find online through some research of your own.

Online sources of information

Knowledge is reassurance: learning more about self-harm can help demystify it, make it seem less frightening, and teach you that you are not alone with this otherwise upsetting and isolating problem.

Everyone should be taught something about self-harm, much as they should about other common life challenges like dealing with drugs and alcohol and feeling in control of their sexual behaviour and health. Talking about self-harm does not somehow make it an acceptable thing to do and therefore more likely to happen, which is what people mean when they say they are worried about *normalising* self-harm, especially among younger people.

If you put 'self harm' into an online search engine, you can quickly find some useful sources of information – for example from NHS Choices and the Royal College of Psychiatrists, or from mental health charities like MIND and the Mental Health Foundation. Their information is worth a read and you will notice some similarities with suggestions and advice in this book.

But ... if you keep searching you may get more confused. Different sites use the terms differently, for example using 'self-harm' to mean only 'self-cutting'. Or they say something like 'People who self-harm are not suicidal'.

I told my GP that I had been looking online about self-harm and I was really confused. What she said was really helpful. She said 'Don't worry – think of it as being like listening in on lots of conversations. Some people seem very confident but are only stating their own opinions and giving a distorted picture, some people are sensible and know what they are talking about. If you read around you can pick up what everybody agrees on and you can find the comments that seem to be accurate about you. We can talk about the rest.'

Trevor, 21

It's fair to say that there is only one real difference of opinion among the sensible people who know what they are talking about – and that's about the idea of *non-suicidal self-injury*. I discussed this in Chapter 3. In essence, some academics and clinicians really like this way of thinking about self-harm and others think that it's wrong. But it's just a way of trying to understand a difficult problem, and debate is healthy.

However, it is important to emphasise that this is one topic for which there is no professional disagreement: no one should be encouraged to harm themselves. If you get that advice from anybody, then that person does not have your best interests at heart.

You may find that taking steps to help yourself is all you need, but if it isn't, and you need to seek professional help, don't worry – the time you have spent trying out some of these approaches isn't wasted. In fact, you will find that it will help you to understand what is on offer and to make the best use of it. In the next chapter I will tell you about what you can expect from professional help in the health service.

chapter 8

Getting help from the health service

This chapter will look at the three parts of the health service that you are most likely to encounter when you seek help for self-harm: the general practice or local health centre where you are registered; the emergency department of an acute hospital; and your local mental health service. In each place you will meet doctors, nurses and perhaps other healthcare professionals. Here are two pieces of advice to start with.

First, don't assume that every health professional that you meet knows much about self-harm and what to do about it. Although self-harm is a really common problem, there are some professionals who have not been trained in the latest ideas about how best to help. So by reading this book you may already know more than they do.

Second, be ready to find that some of the professionals you meet may not behave in a very sympathetic or helpful way. Of course, you may have discovered this already. Why does it happen? One reason is that some people are simply like that: there are health professionals who are only interested in the practical or physical side of health-care and don't have any patience for the emotional side of care. That's improving over time but is never guaranteed.

Another perhaps more surprising reason is this: however upset and frightened you are, you may also be a bit unsettling for a doctor or nurse who is dealing with you. You may make them feel some agitation. They are trying to understand what you have done to yourself and are worried about you and about whether, for example, you might be at risk of suicide. Of course, professionals shouldn't let their own feelings get in the way of offering good care but I must acknowledge that some of them do, especially if their job is generally stressful and they don't have enough time as can happen in an overstretched service. This is doubly bad news because you are probably already sensitive to feeling criticised or ignored, and it would be easy to misread or react strongly to any actions of others that reinforce how you feel. Sometimes a worried professional might seem more focused on how they feel themselves than they are on you.

The point to remember is that your interaction isn't influenced entirely by you – it's also affected by the healthcare professional as an individual. Don't let a negative response from one particular person colour your view of the whole service.

Going to your general practitioner

A typical appointment with a GP is eight to ten minutes. You want to get the best out of that time and your GP wants to be able to make the best decision they can for you. Preparation helps. Here are some tips about what you can do to be ready for the appointment.

1. *Decide if you want to take somebody with you*

   The advantage of going with a person you trust is that they can give you emotional and practical support. Emotionally, they can be there if you get upset. Practically, they may be able to remember details you have forgotten and can afterwards remind you what the doctor said. If you decide to go with someone, you might ask them to make notes about what happens so you can discuss it later. It's your decision if you want to go into the doctor's consulting room with somebody there for support. If you do, you need to check with your supporter that they are happy with this arrangement. Your doctor will also want to know that you are happy for the consultation to be shared with your supporter, because they cannot share information about you with a third party unless they have your consent.

   You can go into the doctor's room on your own if you like, and your supporter can wait outside for you. Of course, anyone can go to see the GP on their own. If you are aged under 16 the doctor will see you but will encourage you to come with a parent or guardian. There are certain treatments they won't give you without your parent's permission.

2. *Decide what you want to say*

   It is always a good idea to have a clear plan and, even if it's really simple, to write it down. Otherwise there's a risk that you will get flustered and forget something. You don't want to leave the room until you have asked the most important questions. There should be at least three points in your plan, so check that you get answers to these questions. The GP really won't mind you checking your notes, and your friend could prompt you. You could even ask them to help you write the list.

◆ What do I want to say? What are the main things I must remember to tell my GP?

◆ What do I want to ask? For example, is there something I've heard about or read about (for example online) that I don't understand or that's worrying me?

◆ What do I want my GP to do? Of course, your GP may not agree with you about the best course of action, or may not be able to do what you want, but she or he will want to know what you want.

Here's a list made by Mary before she went to see her GP for the first time without her mother:

List for my GP visit

Tell her:

I've been doing it secretly for two years.

I feel sad even when I'm playing with Michelle [Mary's younger sister].

I don't like the way my stepdad looks at me.

Ask her:

How can I hide the scar on my thigh?

What help I want:

Can I see somebody to talk to but not a psychiatrist because Tracy sees one and I'm not like her? [Tracy is an acquaintance at college]

---

3. *Be prepared for what your GP will ask*

What your GP will ask is likely to depend on how well they know you already. You can be fairly sure that there are a number of topics they will want to cover, maybe not at a first appointment, but as part of judging how to help you:

◆ What have you done to harm yourself, and how recently? If you have burned or cut yourself is there a wound that might need treatment? If you have taken tablets what did you take, when, and how many? These questions help your GP decide if you need any immediate physical treatment.

◆ How are you feeling now and how were you feeling at the time of the self-harm – for example, have you felt depressed and tearful, worried or anxious, angry? The GP may ask if you have other more unusual experiences, like hearing voices. They will want to know if you are thinking of self-harming again and if you feel suicidal. These questions help your GP decide if you are mentally unwell and how urgently you might need help.

◆ What problems or stresses are there in your life – at home, at school or work, in relationships? These questions help your GP decide what non-medical help you might need.

4. *Make sure you have an open mind about what happens next*

Recent research has shown that when a GP sees

somebody who has self-harmed, they usually do not refer them to a mental health specialist. Why is that? One reason is that many services are underfunded and have what seem like very long waiting times to see non-urgent cases. Some mental health services will only see people who have a diagnosis of mental illness and they don't count self-harm as something they will treat without such a diagnosis. Some psychological therapy services won't treat anybody that they think has a risk of suicide. So GPs get used to managing most problems themselves, unless there is a voluntary organisation that is near where you live that offers help to people who self-harm. You need to be ready for this possibility and to plan with your GP what you are going to do together about your problems.

On the other hand, if your GP does want to refer you then don't say 'No' just because the thought of mental health services frightens you.

I was so not going to psychiatry. I thought all they did was offer you drugs and I heard that if you don't want to take them they just section you. Actually, when I went I was really nervous but it wasn't that bad – we met a couple of times and now I am on a waiting list for therapy, which feels OK.

Charlotte, 18

Maybe you were referred to a mental health specialist or therapist in the past and it didn't help. It is always worth giving something another try – the professional you see is likely to be different and you yourself may well approach the service differently.

In this situation your GP will probably not be keen on prescribing medication for you – and especially not tranquillisers or sleeping tablets. You might consider that tablets would help but, in the longer term, they are more likely to cause you problems than prove beneficial. If you have been low in mood for several weeks or longer, your GP may suggest that you take antidepressant medication. If you are apprehensive don't just say no – ask questions and discuss the advantages and disadvantages. Most importantly, check how long a course of treatment will be and how you will decide when to stop – either because it hasn't worked or because you feel better.

Going to a hospital emergency department

You are likely to go to the emergency department because you need physical treatment for the consequences of something you have recently done to harm yourself – for example, if you're worried that you have taken tablets that might harm you and you want to have an antidote, or if you have a cut that won't stop bleeding or is infected, or you are worried about scarring or other harms.

On the other hand, if you do not need physical treatment then be aware that an acute hospital emergency department (also known as A&E, for Accidents and Emergencies) is not the best place to go for urgent mental healthcare. It is busy, with a high turnover of patients some of whom require very fast and intensive interventions because they are extremely ill physically. There is rarely time or space to evaluate carefully for any complicated psychological problems – especially in the current climate where financial limitations make it hard for emergency departments to respond to increasing pressures.

What to expect in the emergency department

When you arrive, you will have to give information about yourself to a reception member of staff. They ask questions about your name, age and address, and other things that don't seem urgent but that are important. If you are unable to speak, someone can answer these questions for you as much as they are able to. This process is often called 'booking in'.

Once you have booked in you are likely to be seen quickly by a triage nurse who will make a rapid assessment and decide how urgently you need to be seen. The triage nurse is qualified to spot patients who are in a dangerous physical condition, for example their heart is about to stop or they might bleed to death, so they need rapid attention. Their decision about you is based upon a judgement about how urgently you need medical treatment. I am afraid it cannot take much account of how upset you are or how quickly you would like to be seen. What that means is that at busy times you may have to wait some time – perhaps hours – to be seen. This isn't about punishing or neglecting you and the staff don't like it either, but they have difficult choices to make about managing workload in a busy environment.

Common worries about going to A&E

You may have one of the several common worries about the experience at the emergency department.

One is being seen as a time-waster.

I've watched that programme on TV about patients in A&E, how ill they are and how busy the A&E team is. I mean, they never show anybody who's taken an overdose or cut themselves do they? Like – the viewers aren't going to be interested in them are they, and neither are the staff.

Martine, 42

Another is being forced to have physical treatment you don't want, like a stomach wash-out, or being forced to see a psychiatrist, or forced to have psychiatric treatment.

My friend said that in A&E at [hospital name] they made her show them all her scars even though it wasn't part of her treatment. She felt embarrassed, like they were just trying to prove a point or looking out of curiosity. Then they said she wasn't allowed to leave until she had seen a psychiatrist even though she said she wanted to go home and didn't want to wait to see a psychiatrist.

Jonathan, 23

If you are worried about going to the emergency department, remember: when you have treatment in this setting, you have the same rights as in all other areas of healthcare. You have a right to be treated with respect and to have your needs met, regardless of why you are there. Most staff understand that and will try to do their best for you. And you must be asked for your consent for anything that is done to you as investigation or treatment and nothing can be done without your consent.

There is one exception to this rule about your consent being needed, which is if you are judged not to be well enough to make a decision. There are two ways in which this can happen.

First, if at the time they see you the doctors think that you don't have the *mental capacity* to make a decision, in other words if they think that you are too ill to understand exactly what is being asked, or to make a logical decision about what you want to do, then they can treat you if it is in your best interests. This situation is quite rare and the same rule is followed in mental health as in any other part of the NHS, so you should expect to be treated exactly the same as you would in any other healthcare setting.

Second, if the doctors think your judgement is impaired because you are, or might be, suffering from a mental disorder, then they can use the Mental Health Act to detain you while they make a fuller assessment. A doctor in the hospital emergency department can't make this decision on their own, they need to involve other professionals who have to agree – usually an approved social worker and another doctor who is independent of the hospital team treating you in the emergency department. If you want to know more about the Mental Health Act, you can look at one of the leaflets produced by mental health charities that explain it in simple terms, or you can look it up on the NHS Choices website (both listed at the back of this book).

Obviously, there is no point in going for help and then not accepting sensible medical advice, so try to do that. But remember: any action taken should be in agreement with you.

When you are seen by a doctor, physical treatment is likely to come first. This might include blood tests and, if you have taken an overdose, a decision about taking an antidote (something to counteract the effect of the drugs); or cleaning, stitching and dressing of any wounds. This book's remit doesn't extend to cover physical treatments, so I won't say more about them here.

What mental healthcare can you expect?

In the NHS, standards for care are set by the National Institute for Health and Care Excellence, usually called NICE for short. Here's a brief version of what NICE says about the mental healthcare you should receive in the acute hospital.

You should:

1. be cared for with compassion and with the same respect and dignity as any service user;

2. have an initial assessment of your physical health, mental state, your social circumstances and your risks of repetition or suicide;

3. receive the monitoring you need while in the healthcare setting;

4. be cared for in a safe physical environment while in the healthcare setting;

5. receive a comprehensive psychosocial assessment that considers your needs, social situation, psychological state, reasons for harming yourself, feelings of hopelessness, depression or other mental health problems and any thoughts of suicide.

Chapter 1 talked about the seriousness of self-harm and the three ways to assess it – physical, social and psychological. Look at item two on this list from NICE. What it says is exactly that – when somebody sees you they should try to assess your physical health, mental health (psychological state) and your social circumstances.

The first four actions on this list are the responsibility of the medical and nursing staff in the emergency department. They are fairly straightforward and are what you would hope to receive from a caring health service. The more detailed assessment mentioned in number five is often arranged by 'referral'. This is the word that healthcare staff use to say that they are passing you over to another specialist team or professional.

The emergency department staff may make a referral for you to a mental health professional who is part of the hospital's self-harm team. We know from recent research that referral for 'comprehensive assessment' (as described in the NICE guideline, point number five above) often doesn't happen.

*The doctor asked me a few questions when I first saw him
– whether I'd done it before, how I felt now, that sort of
thing. When the blood test came back he said it was OK – a
low level so I didn't need a drip or anything – and he said
I could go home. I was a bit surprised but relieved really, I
just wanted to get out, to be honest.*

Susan, 32

Not everybody is relieved by this decision to be
discharged home after a basic assessment. Friends or
family members can find it surprising and alarming
that no specialist mental health assessment is offered,
especially when no aftercare is arranged. How does that
happen?

One reason is that quite a lot of people who go to
the emergency department decide to leave before they
have been seen or fully assessed. They have second
thoughts or get anxious after too long a wait, or decide
they don't want to see a mental health professional.

The other reason is that hospitals don't always
provide the service that NICE says they should.

The pattern is different in different hospitals, but
across the country something like half the people who
attend the emergency department will eventually go
home without having this specialist assessment. If you
have what NICE calls a comprehensive psychosocial
assessment you spend half an hour or so with a trained
professional, talking about the background to your self-
harm and how you feel now.

What happens instead in the many cases where a
comprehensive psychosocial assessment isn't arranged?

Well, people are told they can leave after physical treatment and the brief initial assessment referred to in point two above, which says: 'Have an initial assessment of your physical health, mental state, your social circumstances and your risks of repetition or suicide.'

You can see that point two places an emphasis on risk assessment. This term 'risk assessment' comes up a lot. It consists of asking you a few questions designed to judge whether you are likely either to repeat self-harm or to kill yourself.

Some people don't mind these risk assessment questions but others really don't like them.

I felt like I was just being put through a sausage machine – it's their agenda not yours, isn't it? They're more interested in ticking boxes than in how you're feeling.

Lee, 19

For doctors or nurses to work effectively they need to have a mental list of the right things to do. In this situation, the list is about what they really need to find out to decide if you are likely to be suicidal. This is sensible, but it tends to feel wrong if the doctor or nurse you are talking to doesn't sound as if they are seeing you as an individual, but are, rather, just checking for the sake of it.

You may be wrong to assume that the doctor isn't interested in you just because they may be literally ticking boxes. This is a very good way for them to make sure that they have covered everything properly – it doesn't mean that they don't care. You may be different from anyone else they have seen so experts have made up lists for doctors and nurses of the important things they must take into account when planning your care.

However the problems with risk assessment, when it is badly done, can be illustrated by this common checklist recommended for use in self-harm assessment:

Modified SAD PERSONS scale

The score is calculated from ten Yes/No questions, with points given for each positive answer as follows:

Sex, male: 1 point
Age 15–25 or 59+ years: 1 point
Depression or hopelessness: 2 points
Previous suicidal attempts or psychiatric care: 1 point
Excessive alcohol or drug use: 1 point
Rational thinking loss (psychotic or organic illness): 2 points
Single, widowed or divorced: 1 point
Organised or serious attempt: 2 points
No social support: 1 point
Stated future intent (determined to repeat or ambivalent): 2 points

This score is then mapped on to a risk assessment scale as follows:

0–5: May be safe to discharge (depending upon circumstances)
6–8: Probably requires psychiatric consultation
9+: Probably requires hospital admission

While there is nothing wrong with asking questions about risk, there is often something wrong with the way it's done here, adding up points for positive answers and producing a 'score' that gives a false sense of applying an accurate test to an individual case. Even without use of a scorecard such as this, asking questions about risk can still be done badly:

◆ in a mechanical or unfeeling way, so that you feel processed or humiliated;

◆ by somebody who doesn't understand how limited this sort of risk assessment is and who uses it as the only source of information when making decisions about your care;

◆ instead of, rather than as well as, a more complete assessment of your problems and what help you need.

However, remember – assessing whether you are at risk is important. Its main function should be to keep you safe and that's why NICE encourages it. And it isn't always done badly!

Suppose you *are* referred, and see somebody from a self-harm team. What are they likely to do? Well, the first bit of it is in the fifth point in that earlier NICE list: 'Receive a comprehensive psychosocial assessment that considers your needs, social situation, psychological state, reasons for harming yourself, feelings of hopelessness, depression or other mental health problems and any thoughts of suicide.'

This sounds like a lot to get through and how much you will cover in a single session will vary depending how much you feel able to talk and how much the person who sees you will want to ask about.

What's the purpose of this assessment? The answer is outlined in the last three points on NICE's list explaining the care you should get:

◆ You should have a collaboratively developed risk management plan. That is, you should try to agree plans about what will keep you safe.

◆ You should have a discussion about the potential benefits of psychological interventions specifically structured for people who self-harm. That is, you should be involved in a discussion about whether therapy will help.

◆ If you are being referred to a different mental health professional, you should have a collaboratively developed plan describing how support will be provided during the changeover. That is, you shouldn't be left in limbo, waiting for an appointment with no help until you see somebody else.

In other words, the point of the comprehensive assessment is to start a discussion about what is best for you once you leave the department.

Making sure that your voice is heard

It says in several places in the NICE guidelines that all these assessments and plans, at every stage in your visit to the emergency department, should be made with you, not just about you. But it can be difficult to take part in plans about your health if you feel frightened or upset and you don't understand what is happening.

Try if at all possible to have somebody with you. If you go to the department on your own, then think about whether there's someone you can call while you are waiting to be seen. A companion will make you feel calmer and can help in any contact with the nurses and doctors, if you are finding it difficult to communicate with them. If you don't have a friend or family member to go with you and your visit is planned in advance, then you can consider going with an advocate. An advocate is somebody (usually a volunteer) who can come with you and speak for you, if you tell them what you want them to say. There may be a local advocacy service near you – if there is then you can get the number by looking online or by asking at your GP's surgery or at the hospital.

Here are three tips about how to make this difficult task a little easier:

◆ Try to take your time and answer any questions you are asked. It'll help the whole experience run a bit more smoothly, even if you can't see the point of it all. Slowing down and thinking about the questions can give you a bit of a breather to consider the next and most important point.

◆ You may feel that at the moment it's most important to get across how you feel, but at least as important is to make clear what help you want. If you aren't sure then ask, maybe a question like: 'I feel as if I need somebody to talk to a bit about my problems but I don't know who I should talk to or how that works – what do you suggest?' Just signalling that you want help and don't know how to get it is the start of what NICE means by 'collaborative discussions' – trying to come up with a joint plan about what to do next.

◆ Some people find it really difficult to say anything at all when they get to the hospital – for any number of reasons the words just won't come. If you think that might apply to you, you could write something down before you go, to give to the nurse or doctor who sees you first. Here's an example:

My name is Alice Smith.

I find it really difficult to talk or answer questions when I am this upset. Please understand, I am not just being difficult.

I have cut my arm quite deep and I think it needs stitches.

It hurts and I want some help with the pain.

I have taken some tablets and I am worried they might damage my kidneys.

People you can contact:

My key worker Jane at SafePlaces. Telephone 0123 456 789

My sister Annie 0789 654 3210

I saw a psychiatrist last time I was here. I don't have an appointment to see him and I don't want to be asked to see a psychiatrist while I am here.

It may be that even if you do write a note like this, what happens isn't exactly what you asked for. You can't always decide exactly what happens in the hospital, but you can at least make sure that your wishes are known.

In the next part of this chapter we will look at what to expect if the result of these discussions is an appointment to see somebody in the mental health services. To finish this section, let me be really clear again about one point: there must be more to assessing your needs and an offer of help than a risk assessment followed by an opinion that you are not mentally ill or that you have mental capacity and therefore don't need further help. Here is what the NICE guidelines say:

> the decision to discharge a person without
> follow-up following an act of self-harm should
> not be based solely upon the presence of low risk
> of repetition of self-harm or attempted suicide
> and the absence of a mental illness, because many
> such people may have a range of other social and
> personal problems.
>
> *NICE Clinical Guideline CG16*

What this means is that you can ask to see somebody if you want, not just to talk about risk but to start a discussion about your problems and what you can do about them.

Going to your local mental health service

It may be that you are referred to a local Community Mental Health Team (often called a CMHT for short). If you are a younger person then the equivalent is the Child and Adolescent Mental Health Service (often called CAMHS for short, pronounced CAMS). These teams include psychiatrists, clinical psychologists, psychiatric social workers, psychiatric nurses and often other professionals. Who you see will depend on your problems and on the way that particular local team works. If the hospital self-harm team runs a clinic, they will offer to see you there (although not many hospitals have such clinics so it is unlikely).

What the mental health team will do is to start with an assessment that is quite like the assessments outlined above, but more detailed. That is, they will assess your needs and any risk to you. You may feel that some of this is just going over what you've already been asked, but it is important to do so. Circumstances change, as do people, and it never hurts for a psychiatrist to check how someone is *now*, not just how they were when they were referred.

After this assessment, you should discuss what plan is best for you. This isn't just about stopping self-harm.

Reducing the risk of self-harm and reducing other risks is important, but it's not the only thing that matters. To be honest, I think psychiatric services have got a bit obsessed with risk and risk assessment and focus too much on the self-harm. The aim of our care should be broader than that – we ought to be helping people to improve how they are able to get on in their day-to-day life both socially and at work, to improve their overall quality of life.

Consultant psychiatrist in a
Community Mental Health Team

One part of the plan needs to involve a discussion about whether therapy is a good idea. Therapy needn't be very time-consuming – sometimes it can involve as few as three or four visits, up to about twelve. There are several types of therapy, all with different (sometimes rather silly) names. For now, it's worth saying just a little about what they aim to do. A simple way to look at this is to think there are three main aims of therapy:

1. **Helping you to tackle unhelpful ways of thinking**.
   For example, you may be very self-critical, running yourself down all the time, or untrusting of other people. These ways of thinking may lead you to avoid close relationships and people in general. When you think about your life or the past you tend to concentrate on the negatives. Or maybe you are impulsive and not very flexible in the way you tackle problems.
   The best-known therapy that takes the approach of tackling your thinking is one you may have heard of: CBT. The 'C' stands for 'cognitive', which means 'ways of thinking'; the 'B' stands for 'behavioural', which means 'and how it affects what you do'. 'T' is for therapy. Typically, therapy involves spending time identifying your own personal style of thinking and how it is related to what you do (that is, the way

you behave). For example, if you habitually assume that people don't like you, then you may turn down invitations to go out and miss the opportunity to meet new people or discover that people do like you (and that's why you got the invitation!). You can then work with a therapist to challenge the way you think, and to try new and different activities in your life to see what effect they have. CBT varies in length; a typical session lasts 45 to 50 minutes and you may be offered a few sessions first as a trial. Sometimes (but not very often) therapy may go on for sixteen to eighteen sessions, but usually it is more like six or eight.

A more intensive and longer therapy with similar aims is Dialectical Behaviour Therapy. It is like CBT in some ways, but DBT can also involve group therapy and sometimes social skills training, to tackle problems you feel you have interacting with other people.

2. **Helping you to find new ways to tackle the problems that cause your self-harm**. We saw earlier how difficulties with problem-solving were common in people who self-harm, so it's not surprising that there's a type of therapy called 'problem-solving therapy' that aims to teach you new ways of building skills in this area. The steps of problem-solving are outlined in Chapter 6.

Because so many of life's important problems are in relationships, therapies that help you think about relationships are worth considering. Sometimes they are called interpersonal therapies

– interpersonal means 'between people'. One example is Psychodynamic Interpersonal Therapy (PIT for short). These therapies explore what is going wrong in your relationships and what you might be able to do to change the ways you relate to other people – for example, exploring why you find trust difficult and how unhelpful it can be to avoid closeness to others as your preferred way of dealing with mistrust.

It may be that going to therapy as a couple or with your family in 'family therapy' is the best way to help; this is common in CAMHS services. In therapy, family can include anybody who acts as a parent, brother or sister or child – even if they aren't your biological relative. The definition of 'family' in this setting is that you live together in a way that should be mutually supporting.

3. **Helping you decide what your goals and values in life are, and do better at achieving them**. These therapies are interesting because instead of concentrating on the problems you have, they concentrate on more positive aspects of your life and help you to work out how you can build on those. One example is what's called Acceptance and Commitment Therapy (ACT for short).

Not all these therapies are available everywhere, but most are. The NHS can provide the common therapies noted above and you can ask about what is available locally and how you can access it – whether you need a referral, for example by your GP, or whether you can make contact directly yourself with a therapy service.

part four

What else do I need to know?

chapter 9

When you don't get the healthcare you want

There's no point in denying it – people who self-harm do not always find that their experience of healthcare is a good one. The commonest complaints about services are that the patient as an individual is treated poorly; that compulsory treatment is threatened; or that there is a failure to offer any treatment at all.

Poor treatment of me as a person

It is unforgivable that it is still possible to hear of people being spoken to rudely or dismissively.

The nurse who saw me first just said to me 'Not you again, haven't you got something better to do than to keep coming in here?' I wanted to sink through the floor and at the same time I felt angry – I mean, it's not as if I do it just to pass the time of day.

> Jess, 26, about her third attendance
> in the emergency department

These attitudes and behaviours aren't just rude or insensitive, they are bad healthcare because they contribute to the problem that the responsible health professional is supposed to be addressing – and they shouldn't be tolerated.

Sometimes the rudeness or lack of consideration is less open than that. It can take the form of insensitivity in asking personal questions in a space that isn't private – like a cubicle in the emergency department with just a curtain pulled across.

You might think that it's a doctor's job to examine you, but you might also wonder why they need to look at old scars when it doesn't make any difference to the treatment you are going to get now.

The doctor insisted on me taking my top off so she could 'examine me properly'. I couldn't see why ... I'd told her what I'd done in the past and it was only the new cut I was worried about. It was just awful. And then somebody else walked in and they started talking about somebody else's tests just as if I wasn't there ... as if 'Oh she's just a cutter, she doesn't matter.'

Jude, 35

Remember that you have to give consent for any examination or treatment given to you, and that consent has to be informed. So it is perfectly reasonable to ask why you are being asked to do something if you can't see why it is a part of your treatment, and to decline to give consent if you aren't offered a sensible explanation for what is proposed.

Threats about compulsory treatment

Hospital emergency departments seem to vary considerably in the way they treat people who go there after self-harm. Some are brilliant and do the best they can for everybody, regardless of why they are there. A few, I'm afraid, don't offer such a good experience. Many offer a service that is variable in standard, and can offer a good experience on one occasion and a poor one on another.

One aspect of care that I've heard complaints about is the use of threats (at least, that is how they are experienced) of coercion.

After I'd had the wound treated I said I wanted to go home and they said I couldn't until I had seen the duty psychiatrist. I said I didn't want to but they said I had to – they'd call security to stop me if I tried to leave.

Charlie, 27

Of course there can be worrying situations where, as a health professional, you don't want someone to leave without a proper assessment of how suicidal they are. This approach, of insisting that a patient stays, sometimes seems to be applied as a blanket policy rather than decided on case by case. That isn't right – the law is clear that a person must be assumed to have mental capacity unless there is evidence to doubt it, so consent is needed for all healthcare unless there are grounds to invoke either the Mental Capacity Act or the Mental Health Act.

Failure to offer mental health treatment

We've already discussed in this book that people who self-harm aren't always offered expert help with their mental health problems:

◆ Fewer than a third of GP visits at which self-harm is noted are followed by a referral for mental healthcare.

◆ In fewer than half of cases of self-harm seen in a general hospital is a psychosocial assessment made or aftercare arranged – most commonly the patient is advised to go and see their GP.

◆ Mental health services concentrate on what they call 'severe mental illness', which doesn't include self-harm.

I saw a psychiatric nurse in my local Community Mental Health Team. She said that because I wasn't a suicide risk they wouldn't be offering me treatment. She suggested I called Samaritans if I felt like harming myself again.

Erin, 26

What can you do about poor care?

First, as always, think about prevention. That's why it is best, if possible, to take someone with you to any visits about your healthcare. There are two issues here – in general you are less likely to be treated badly if you are accompanied. And that can help if you're not in the best shape to represent your own interests. In a crisis, it's easy to clam up or to get angry, or you may be someone who drinks to help symptoms, or you may have taken tablets that affect your mental state. For all those reasons, another voice to support yours may be helpful.

There may be a local advocacy service near you – if

there is then you can get the number by looking online or by asking at your GP's surgery or at the hospital.

If you decide you want to say something about being badly treated, you don't necessarily have to make a formal complaint. You can ask to speak to someone or you can write to somebody to express your concerns and ask them to look into it. Many services appreciate this sort of feedback.

◆ At your GP, there will be a Patient Group, sometimes called a Patient Reference Group. Reception staff can give you details. Or you can contact the Practice Manager directly.

◆ In a hospital, you can contact the nurse in charge of the department where you were seen, or the nurse in charge of the ward, or the matron. Hospitals have a Patient Advice and Liaison Service (PALS) that, as the name suggests, should be able to offer advice about what to do.

Suppose you decide that you do want to take it further and make a formal complaint. Every NHS organisation has a complaints procedure. It should be easy to find on their website, on signs in their premises, or by asking a member of staff. In hospitals, the process is managed at a senior level so that you don't have to deal directly with the team who have treated you and might treat you again. In general practice, there is an organisation called the Clinical Commissioning Group (CCG) that handles complaints. These organisations have a responsibility to make sure that:

- ◆ Your complaint is dealt with efficiently, properly and within a stated period of time.
- ◆ You will be told the outcome of the investigation of your complaint.
- ◆ You are clear what to do next if you aren't happy with the way your complaint was handled.
- ◆ You are informed about the possibilities for compensation if you have been harmed by your treatment.

The mental health charities listed at the end of this book may also be able to offer you advice.

chapter 10

Self-harm in society – additional topics

Self-harm is a very personal matter – it is closely related to our emotional and mental health, and typically arises as a response to troubles in our personal world. So why is there a chapter in this book about 'self-harm and society'?

There are two reasons for this chapter. The first is to discuss social stereotypes about who self-harms – and especially to challenge the idea that self-harm is always done by young women with personality problems. These stereotypes come from society. And the second is to ask what steps can be taken in wider society to help reduce the frequency of self-harm; that is, to make it less likely that it's something people want to do when they have troubles or stresses in their lives.

Self-harm and social attitudes

Sometimes it seems as if self-harm is always in the news. It alarms and concerns people, and it also appears to fascinate us. It is worldwide. Under the headline '"Soaring" numbers of under-16s admitted to hospital for self-harming', the *Independent* newspaper reported that:

The overwhelming majority of children were taken in because they had tried to poison themselves with drugs, alcohol, pesticides, household solvents and other toxic substances ... Others, including some aged between five and nine, had tried to hang themselves. The figures also showed that children aged between one and five were among the youngsters that needed treatment.

Independent, 5 April 2016

We ask ourselves – what's wrong that so many people want to harm themselves? Perhaps this question is particularly uncomfortable when we ask why self-harm is so common among younger people, who ought to be looking forward to life.

I want to touch on several topics that come up when I discuss this topic of self-harm in society, and the first is the question of gender.

Self-harm and gender

When I worked in acute hospital medicine in the 1970s, each medical team took a turn at being on duty for a day of admitting medical emergencies. It was very rare that a 'duty day' went by without us admitting two or three people who needed medical treatment for a drug overdose. It was striking even then how many of these patients were young women. In fact in the 1960s and 1970s, women outnumbered men by three or four to one in most hospitals. As I noted in Chapter 2, this pattern is still obvious today, decades later, although not as extreme. Why is that? There is no biological reason why young women should be more at risk of self-harm, so it must be something about their lives. If it is, then should we see self-harm as a feminist issue?

The key to answering this question lies in the fact that self-harm only really becomes common after puberty. There are demands on girls and young women in their teenage years that are about pressure to conform or fit in. There are whole industries built around making women worry about how they look – their weight, what shape their bodies are, what clothes they wear – and it's not difficult to see how powerful these influences are on girls during the years when their bodies are changing and they are starting to make adult relationships.

When I was 14 I just used to spend hours looking at pictures in magazines and thinking – 'I don't look like that, nobody will ever find me attractive, my thighs are too fat and my breasts aren't the right size for the rest of me. It was like – I don't like my body, and my body is me, so how can anybody like me?'

Josie, 23

Coupled with this pressure to conform in how you look and dress, there's a pressure to fit in socially – in how you behave in relationships, both romantic and otherwise. This might be described as a need to be liked. You might think that being likeable isn't a bad thing, but what if being liked doesn't come just from having likeable characteristics (being kind, or funny or loyal) but from doing what other people (and especially boys) want? There's a lot in the media that focuses on peer pressure and its relation to girls' sexual behaviour, and that's important. But it goes wider – if you only feel liked or valued for the way you respond to the expectations of others, then your other relationships are also affected: with friends, teachers, colleagues, strangers. You can't feel relaxed and be yourself if you are always trying to project an image or fit in with what somebody else wants – it makes young women vulnerable to feelings of rejection and failure when relationships break up, and that's a common story about what leads up to self-harm.

After he finished with me I just felt so … I don't know, as if there was nothing for me. I couldn't believe he'd do it, I'd trusted him completely and he said he loved me and I believed that. Now I think – what did I do wrong? I don't know who to trust, I just can't be hurt like that again.

Lorna, 17

Given all these considerations, we can say: 'Yes, self-harm is a feminist issue.' This isn't to conclude that there is nothing to be said about men and self-harm, simply that higher rates among girls and young women need to be explored and explained. We will then be in a stronger position to offer specific help for young women who self-harm. At the moment it can feel as if there is a fair bit of bemoaning the content of social media and its effect on young women, and then, when it comes to psychological help, gender takes a back seat.

For men there are different pressures, the most

obvious being the expectations of masculine behaviour. These expectations mirror those on girls but the emphasis is very different. There are, of course, any number of pictures of men in magazines – effortlessly stylish, implausibly muscular – but they aren't as overwhelmingly defining of what men should be as are the images of women. Perhaps more important than how men look are expectations of how men should behave – being dominant, taking the lead – which create their own pressures.

From a young age, boys are discouraged from showing emotion. You might think that this is changing when you see pictures of footballers crying after losing an important game, or when a high-profile adult talks about the effect on them of the death of a loved one. But it is still true that emotional expression isn't as widely expected in young men – how many feel comfortable crying in front of others because they are lonely, or because a relationship has finished?

Another feature of masculinity that is important here is the male tendency to aggression. In the same way that men are more likely to be involved in violence, they are more likely to do violent things to themselves. This certainly seems to be a factor in the higher rates of suicide among men than women – men are more likely to kill themselves by violent means such as hanging or jumping from a height while women die more often by self-poisoning.

In summary, gender is always relevant in self-harm. As a friend or family member, or as a practitioner, it is always worth considering what gender-related aspects are important, and worth asking about them in a sympathetic way.

Self-harm and ethnicity

Is self-harm something that only white people do? You might think so, from most of what is written about it. The truth is that no one knows quite how common self-harm is in other ethnic groups. There are exceptions and several research studies, for example, have shown that self-harm is common among young women of Asian and particularly South Asian heritage. By comparison we know very little about young men of Asian heritage. They don't present to health services often, but we don't know if that's because self-harm is rarer or because they don't want to seek help in this way.

There are several reasons why we don't know much about ethnicity and self-harm. One problem is that routine recording of ethnicity is so unreliable in health records. Research studies sometimes use quite crude categories for ethnicity, for example lumping all 'Asian' people together. Patterns can change quite quickly. For example many of the younger women seen after self-harm fifteen or twenty years ago were children of first-generation immigrants whereas young women now are more likely to have grown up in a family with parents who are British by birth.

Another reason is that people from minority ethnic groups are more reluctant to use services for mental health problems. It is often said that different ethnic groups have different experiences of mental health problems and mental health services and that one explanation might be institutional racism, where services don't understand how to provide services that reflect cultural and other needs. So, people don't want to engage with a service that might misdiagnose or wrongly treat them.

What we do know about self-harm is that even in minority ethnic groups, the reasons for it are pretty much the same as outlined in earlier parts of this book. The main differences occur in families with a history of recent immigration, where attitudes in older generations can cause tension with members of younger generations.

I grew up in England and I think of myself as British, and I'm a Muslim and my parents still call Pakistan home. I don't have a problem with any of that, but sometimes I have a problem with the things that go with it. I want to choose my own friends and who I go out with, and I don't want to have to answer my mum's questions all the time about what I'm doing. It makes me angry and then we have rows.

Fatima, 19

If this experience of tension at home is coupled with experiences of racism and rejection outside the home, then it's easy to see how isolation and unhappiness can develop, with a sense of not quite belonging anywhere leading to difficulty in imagining where help might lie.

When I came here with my family, it felt as if we'd be safe at last – no more fighting and not knowing if you'd be safe when you went out. But I get loads of trouble on the street

and called Paki and that, and even in the news it's all on
about immigrants who shouldn't be here and I'm frightened
of being sent to an immigration centre.

Rasheed, 16, refugee from Syria

Talking about self-harm – words and stigma

The words we use to describe people reflect our attitudes to those people. 'Stigma' means, literally, a mark, and when we use words that mark people out as different, outsiders in some way, and undesirable, then we are stigmatising them.

There are several reasons why self-harm is stigmatised. Because the harm is self-inflicted it is seen as undeserving of the sympathy that would be granted if it had been the result of an attack or an accident. The reasons behind it are dismissed; it is associated with being a woman in a gender-biased society; some think it is caused by a personality abnormality; and it isn't seen as 'treatable' and is therefore a waste of professionals' time.

There are two behaviours that follow from the way society stigmatises self-harm: labelling the people who do it; and describing their reasons for self-harm in a dismissive way.

You will sometimes hear terms like 'cutter' or 'self-harmer' used to describe people. In my experience, such terms are more frequently used to describe women. This way of talking may not be intended deliberately to cause offence: after all it seems merely to describe what a person has done. But that's the point – labelling someone for what they do is like saying: 'This is what defines who you are and there's nothing else I really need to say about you.' Like labelling people addicted to drugs as 'druggies', the label makes it harder to see behind the behaviour to the person. It is dismissive and offensive and it should be avoided.

Apart from demeaning the individual, labelling can belittle their reasons for self-harm. It's not uncommon to hear self-harm talked about as 'attention-seeking' or 'manipulative'. This suggests that there is no real distress involved but that the person who self-harms is just making a dramatic gesture for the sake of the effect it has on others. It is certainly true that sometimes people self-harm in the hope that it will change the behaviour of others – leading them to be more caring, or to step in and help. But to acknowledge that should not be to dismiss the act. After all, how desperate does somebody have to be if harming themselves is the best way they can think of to attract attention and care from another person?

Over time, health professionals have moved away from the attitudes reflected in these demeaning labels. One example of that shift in professional thinking is the change in recent times from talking about 'deliberate self-harm' to talking about 'self-harm'. Although the word 'deliberate' was originally used to distinguish it from accidental self-harm (such as drinking poison that had been stored in an unlabelled drinks bottle), it was perceived by some as implying that the motives weren't psychologically important – as if someone had just casually decided, 'I'll harm myself today'. Not everyone has agreed with this renaming, but a general move in that direction is positive, and a sign of how seriously health professionals take the issue of stigmatising language.

Can we prevent self-harm?

This book has presented several times the idea that self-harm is a response to stressful circumstances – that it can't all be put down to psychological problems in the individual. This observation raises the question of whether there are actions that can be taken to change the environment and to make society a different place in an effort to reduce self-harm rates. Below are three types of prevention programmes: schools-based programmes; alcohol and drug policy; and controlling social media.

School-based programmes

Because self-harm starts becoming common at about the time most children are going to secondary school, and because pretty much every child goes to school, it is natural to wonder if it would be possible to do something in schools that made a difference. Such programmes are not universal but are being actively promoted now, and can have three aims:

1. **Teaching children about other ways of dealing with stress and with emotional symptoms.** Self-harm has become so common that it might seem like 'what you do', especially if nobody suggests alternatives.

I was that upset when my dad left I couldn't think ... I didn't know what to do. I was round at Tracey's [a friend] and I found some tablets when I went to the bathroom. I just took them and swallowed them on the way home. I don't know what I was thinking.

Martina, 13

2. **Teaching positive life skills.** Here the approach is more about learning general skills, for example in managing relationships and being assertive without being aggressive.

I used to be like, it was everything he wanted until I couldn't take it no more and then I'd get angry and tell him to get lost. There was nothing in between and I was miserable because either we were rowing or he was getting his way. I've started to learn to be different, in small ways. Now I'll say, 'I want to be with you, but you've got to listen to me sometimes and do what I want' and he is getting better with that too.

Lou, 16

3. **Providing on-site mental health support.** Schools are now being encouraged through government policy to provide students with access to mental health support in school. The idea is to offer the sort of advice and support noted above, and to provide the opportunity for the more severely troubled young people to see a mental health professional. On the other hand, such services need to be properly resourced and their staff should be trained and supported. It won't help if schools point too many

young people towards mental health services, overwhelming those services and causing delays for the small number of seriously concerning young people as well as wasting time for others.

In 2016, the Department for Education provided a 'blueprint' for what counselling in schools in England should be like. It talks about a 'whole school' approach to mental health and well-being. This includes:

◆ approaches to improving well-being and resilience, about which the report says: 'Schools will have a range of activities in place to support this. These range from those with a direct focus on mental wellbeing, for example, using mindfulness techniques, to others which build character and provide emotional fulfilment, for example the Duke of Edinburgh award, music and cultural activities. Other activities encourage teamwork and healthy living, for example, sport and physical activities.'

◆ raising awareness of mental health issues through the curriculum

◆ reducing the stigma around mental health

◆ an effective school pastoral system

◆ leadership and support from the top of the school.

Not all these ideas have much evidence for them and planning is not far advanced for their delivery in most places, so we don't know how effective they can be. All we can say is that the basic principles are sound and that time will tell.

Alcohol and drug policy

Alcohol is too cheap and drugs are too readily available, and both are too readily used as a response to stress.

Consultant psychiatrist, North of England

Everyone seems to have an opinion about national policy on alcohol pricing, the decriminalisation of cannabis, or related issues. It was thought that increasing the cost of alcohol to a minimum of 50p per unit in Scotland might, as the papers said when it was introduced on 1 May 2018, 'curb the nation's drink problem'. Cheap, high-strength, easily available alcohol is a recognised temptation for people on low incomes with big problems. But it was also argued that the price change meant nothing to well-paid people and was just discrimination against the poor.

It is not the place of this book to weigh into those debates. But I do think it is fair to say this: any policy that makes drugs and alcohol more readily available will make them more readily available to everybody, including young people and people with mental health problems. Drug and alcohol use are both associated with self-harm, and stopping the use of alcohol is one of the actions reported as effective by people who have stopped self-harming. So liberalising policy, or failing to introduce more restrictive policy, has the potential to increase risk for those most likely to self-harm. That consequence needs to be taken into consideration in any policy change.

Regulating social media

Social media – the collective of online communication channels that can be accessed on computers and smartphones, such as Facebook, Twitter, Instagram and Snapchat – is a relatively new way of keeping in touch and learning about the world. Pretty much everybody uses social media in some form or another. And yet at the same time we worry about its influence. Social media content is often unreliable or deliberately misleading; you never quite know who you're dealing with when so many users have fictional names and multiple accounts; and content can be offensive or even worse, bullying, pornographic or seductive. Maybe, it is argued, less of this stuff should be available or at least it should be harder for vulnerable people to access. At the same time, we know that young people spend hours of their waking lives accessing social media and the more socially isolated and troubled they are, the more time they seem to spend online.

Even a liberal person who supports free speech is horrified that there are sites apparently dedicated to talking positively about self-harm and some that seem actively to encourage people to do it.

What evidence would support a policy to regulate social media? First, we need to know what the cause-and-effect relationship is between social media use and mental health problems. That is, does social media use cause mental health problems and ideas of self-harm, or is it that people who have mental health problems tend to use social media more than most? And second, we need to know what use people make of social media when they do have mental health problems. Might they in fact be using these sites, whatever an outsider thinks of their content, as a source of support in the sense that engaging with the site relieves them and reduces their urge to act, rather than strengthening it?

The answer to the first of these questions is that it almost certainly works both ways. Young people who are unhappy and isolated tend to spend more time online, and spending a great deal of time online isn't a great way to get out of a rut in your thinking and build the sort of life that will make you happier.

Research offers some idea about how people use social media, both from asking them directly and from looking at the content of posts. What we learn is that quite a lot of social media activity by those who self-harm is not about self-harm at all, it's just chatting about the more or less trivial things that most people chat about most of the time – clothes, music, sport and so on.

When self-harm is the topic, then the commonest posts simply share the experience of the poster – distress, or frustration or anger. Sometimes the language used is quite like the language of addiction: 'It's something I want to stop but keep coming back to.' Occasionally there are supportive comments. Active encouragement to undertake self-harm is rare.

Interesting research undertaken at the Institute of Health Sciences in Leeds sheds a different light on this question. One of our students studied over 600 posts on three popular social media sites, all of which had been tagged 'self harm'. What she found suggested that a more complicated conversation was going on, with two main topics other than self-harm: what we might term 'experiencing the body' and 'belonging and not belonging'.

'Experiencing the body' included a variety of texts and images about body image and being thin, accompanied by cartoons, photographs and drawings of a whole range of bodies. As researchers we were struck by how many were of uncertain gender, as if the poster (the person posting the images) was breaking away from simple male–female distinctions. We know that worries about sexuality and gender roles are common concerns of young people, and while such worries weren't stated explicitly in the posts it seemed that these concerns were an underlying theme.

'Belonging and not belonging' included posts about trust and relationships, meeting the expectations of others, what it means to be glamorous or attractive, and how much to show who you really are or to put on a front.

In summary, I think we can say a couple of things about social media. First, most of its content doesn't suggest that it is likely to be harmful, but more that it provides a means for people to explore dilemmas in their lives and to express emotions in a safe way that doesn't impinge too directly on those close to them.

That said, trying to limit the amount of time spent online is a good thing for other reasons – because such preoccupation with online life limits physical activity and because it is socially isolating in the sense that it doesn't involve face-to-face contact in the real world.

What about those rare sites that actively recommend or encourage self-harm or suicide? Should they be banned? We don't know how much, if at all, they lead people to self-harm or if they have the opposite effect by confronting the challenge head-on. My personal opinion is that they probably don't do as much harm as people think, but I don't believe either that they do any good. You might consider that the world wouldn't be worse off if they were banned and that such a small step would not do any damage to our right of free speech while it might make a few people safer. Other people might think that banning these sites would be the thin end of the wedge.

Resources and helpful organisations

In this list, I am not making recommendations about any of the organisations named. I am simply offering contact details and suggesting that you might like to try getting it touch with them for advice, information about local contacts, or for more information about self-harm and what you can do.

24-hour telephone services

These numbers were correct at the time of going to press.

- Your GP's number will divert to the 24-hour service out of hours
- **NHS 24** Tel: 111
- **Samaritans** – a voluntary support organisation for anyone feeling suicidal

Tel: 116 123 (24-hour service)
Email jo@samaritans.org
Freepost RSRB-KKBY-CYJK, PO Box 9090, STIRLING, FK8 2SA

Other voluntary organisations

Childline – for children and young people under 19
childline.org.uk
Tel. 0800 1111 – the number won't show up on your phone bill

Harmless
harmless.org.uk
1 Beech Avenue, Nottingham NG7 7LJ

info@harmless.org.uk
Harmless is a user-led organisation that provides a range of services including support, information, training and consultancy to people who self-harm, their friends and families, and professionals and those at risk of suicide.

Papyrus UK – a voluntary organisation for people under 35
papyrus-uk.org

- Provides confidential help and advice to young people and anyone worried about a young person
- Helps others to prevent young suicide by working with and training professionals
- Campaigns and influences national policy

Tel. Hopeline UK 0800 068 41 41 – Monday to Friday 10am to 10pm, weekends 2pm to 10pm, bank holidays 2pm to 5pm
Text 07786 209697
Email pat@papyrus-uk.org

Rethink Mental Illness – support for all aspects of mental health, including advice about self-harm
rethink.org

Selfharm UK – particularly for young people who self-harm
selfharm.co.uk

Self-injury support (formerly Bristol Crisis Service for Women)
selfinjurysupport.org.uk
All services open Tuesday, Wednesday, Thursday 7pm to 9.30pm
Tel: 0808 800 8088
Text 07537 432444
Email info@selfinjurysupport.org.uk

The Silver Line – for older people
thesilverline.org.uk
Tel: 0800 470 8090

Young Minds – supporting all aspects of mental health need for young people, including advice about self-harm
youngminds.org.uk
Text <YM> to 85258
Parents' helpline: 0808 802 5544 (Monday to Friday, 9.30am–4.00pm)

Other sources of information

MIND

mind.org.uk
In addition to its role as a mental health charity, MIND produces information on a range of mental health topics including the Mental Health Act:
mind.org.uk/media/3444972/mental-health-act-1983_2016.pdf

NHS Choices

nhs.uk/conditions/self-harm
Offers information and advice on a wide range of health problems. A useful alphabetical index can be searched for any physical or mental health problem.

NICE Guidelines

There are two sets of guidelines, on the short-term management and the longer-term management. They are written for professionals, but there are accessible versions for the general public:
nice.org.uk/guidance/cg16/informationforpublic
nice.org.uk/guidance/cg133/ifp/chapter/About-this-information

Royal College of Psychiatrists

rcpsych.ac.uk/expertadvice/problems/depression/self-harm.aspx
The Royal College of Psychiatrists is a professional body that supports psychiatrists practising in the UK and also provides educational and informational materials for patients.

Acknowledgements

I was pleased to respond when my long-time colleague Professor June Andrews asked me if I would write a book about self-harm in the One Stop series. I am grateful to her for the encouragement to do so, and for the excellent model she provided me in her own book in the same series, on dementia.

My colleagues Lou Pembroke, Russell Pembroke and David Owens were generous in the time they gave to reading drafts of the manuscript and making comments. It was helpful to receive professional feedback and comments from two other clinical and academic experts in the field, professors Else Guthrie and Nav Kapur. Jacqui Morrissey and her colleagues at Samaritans kindly also provided their insightful views.

I have worked with many clinicians over the years, from nursing, psychiatry, social work and allied health professions. We have shared an interest in people who self-harm and what we can do to help, and I have learned much from them – as of course I have from the many people who have been personally affected by self-harm who have shared their experiences with me.

Finally, the meticulous reading of Louisa Dunnigan and Susanne Hillen at Profile provided me with many useful comments and suggestions from the perspective of an independent reader.

Having offered all my genuine thanks, it remains only to remind you that of course the views expressed in this book are my own, and that any errors of fact or of judgement – are entirely my responsibility.

Starting on page 181, I offer a list of resources that I hope, like this book, you will find useful, and will encourage you to learn more about and understand the important problem of self-harm. This isn't an academic book and there are no academic references in it, but if you want to know more I will be happy to try to provide you with details. You can write by email to OneStopSelfHarm@gmail.com. I cannot, of course, comment on personal or individual cases or circumstances, but if you disagree with something I have said or think I have made a mistake, do let me know – I am always learning.

Index